ICE WATER
PLEASE

My Life as a Proud Alcoholic and a Formula to Help One Person **Stop Drinking Forever**

EDDIE ARANA

Printed by IngramSpark in the United States of America.
First printing 2021.

www.icewaterplease.com

This is dedicated to my parents, Carlos and Aida Arana, who both passed away during the writing of this book. My biggest fear in life was losing one of you—and I lost both of you within five months. Thank you very much for being the greatest parents any son could ever have. I love both of you so much, and I am sorry for what I put you through.

P.S. I am still sober.

CONTENTS

FOREWORD

I ALMOST DIED because of my drinking habit. I lost my family because of my drinking. Everything that I valued and loved was almost lost because of my drinking. So, after many years and tries, I developed a formula and eventually stopped drinking.

"Eddie, you have to write a book."

I have heard this said hundreds of times from all kinds of people. I hate writing. However, I enjoy the finished product of writing, and I enjoy the responses from people that my writing brings out. About ten years ago, I started writing daily "Drinking Stories" posts on Facebook from July 1 through July 15 to culminate on and commemorate my sobriety date of July 15, 2004 (as of this writing—hopefully it is still my sobriety date when you are reading this). Every year, I would write fifteen new stories. The truth is, I enjoy reminiscing about my drinking days. They were fun—a lot of fun. I cannot deny that. Unfortunately, all of that fun caught up with me. It eventually all backfired on me.

I first started drinking in 1979 when I was sixteen years old—and twenty-five years later, I became sober. Along the way, some pretty funny shit happened to me. This book is a truthful account of my adventures, feelings, and experiences. I always wished some asshole could have written a book like this when I was growing up; it would have saved me a lot of stress, money, and embarrassment. I am ashamed of the things that I did when I was drunk, but the shame does not make those stories any less entertaining.

This book will cover my days as a drinker—funny stories about my drinking, not-so-funny stories about my drinking—as well as my road to sobriety. I believe I have a winning formula to stop drinking, and I hope to teach it to at least one other person. My goal is to help others with their drinking problems, and I will be extremely happy if I succeed. Getting sober isn't the most glamorous experience; however, it will save your life.

I hope my story helps you.
Good luck!

THE WORST AND BEST NIGHT OF MY LIFE

July 15, 2004

I WAS STRAPPED down in a hospital bed at Lutheran General Hospital in Park Ridge, Illinois, and dying to urinate. I was yelling for the nurse to help me because I was in a straitjacket situation and I couldn't move my arms. I had to piss! The nurse offered me a bottle to urinate in. Thank God. When she pulled away my hospital gown, she discovered a lime-green condom on my penis (the glow-in-the-dark kind). I had to do some quick thinking, and I said to her in a half-joking manner, "Oh, those jokers at the club." She just shook her head, gave me that look (and we all know what kind of look she gave me—the look of a disappointed and rather angry maternal figure), removed the condom, and let me take my piss. That was it. That situation was the end result of twenty-five years of drinking. This was my rock bottom. I was scared.

On July 15, 2004, I was forty-one years old and married to my wife, T. C., with three kids—Sarah, my oldest daughter, was ten; little Eddie, my son, who was eight; and Isabelle, my youngest daughter, who was three.

How had I gotten here? How had my life become so bad that I ended up in a hospital room with a condom on my penis and no recollection of how it got there? What the fuck was wrong with me? T. C. was already on her way to the hospital—what was I going to say to her about this one?

God, help me think of an excuse to get me out of this one, I prayed. I promise you that if you help me this final time, I will never drink again. Fuck, she's here! Please don't be in a bad mood. Please feel sorry for me. Please nurture me. Please don't make me stop drinking. Please don't tell my parents. Please don't tell the kids. Fuck, fuck, fuck . . .

The evening started off innocently enough with a Chicago Cubs rooftop party across the street from Wrigley Field. Max Waisvisz, owner of the rooftop, had invited me over to have a few drinks. I very rarely took my car whenever I went out drinking, but this particular night, I broke my own rule and drove. I arrived at the rooftop around 6 p.m. and had about seven or eight Miller Lite beers. Of the twenty-five times I have been to a Wrigley Field rooftop party, I do not believe I have seen a single pitch being thrown. I was there strictly for the drinking. I knew a bunch of friends at the party and was having a relatively good time, but I was uncomfortable about having my car with me and drinking and driving. I had a major fear of getting a DUI.

At about 9 p.m., I left for Zia's Trattoria in Edison Park on the Northwest Side of Chicago, where I met up with three guys whom I knew from the neighborhood. Zia's was about a mile from my house, so I felt a little better about the driving situation. The guys were sitting around the bar area, just laughing it up, and I had about three or four more beers there. I invited a couple of my friends from Zia's to the Park Ridge Country Club where there was a private members event called Plae Day. I was proud to be a member of the Park Ridge Country Club.

I thought it was a very big deal to have had "made it" in life. T. C. had also wanted us to join the country club, though she would come to regret it later. I would consider myself popular there, mostly because of my drinking exploits.

I drove my friends to the country club from Zia's in my 2004 Mercedes Benz E300. The Park Ridge Country Club was located about a block from my house in Park Ridge. The hard alcohol started to flow, and I started drinking Glenlivet single malt scotch—on the rocks. I had at least ten scotches there. Okay, let's add up the drinks—ten to twelve beers and about ten scotches for a total of at least twenty drinks. My last recollection of the night was buying everyone scotches and eventually just passing out on a sofa near the bar.

I left the club around 3 a.m. and got into my car. Keep in mind that I lived about a block from the country club and could have very easily walked home. I do not remember the ride at all. The Park Ridge Fire Department had to pull me out of the car using the "jaws of life." I had totaled my car, totaled another car parked on the street, and taken out a fire hydrant on the lawn in front of a house (and, no, the water from the fire hydrant did not gush out—a very popular question that I always get). Subsequently, I saw pictures of my totaled car, and it was a miracle that I lived through that accident.

The next thing I remember was being in the hospital, wanting to urinate. July 15, 2004, was the date. I will never forget that date because it was the last day that I ever had a drink.

July 15, 2004, was the worst night of my life because I almost died in a car accident and could have very easily killed someone else. July 15, 2004, was also the best night of my life because it made me realize what a fucking moron I was and that I needed to stop drinking completely. I was lucky enough to survive.

It took a great deal of soul searching to finally walk into a bar one day and hear the bartender ask, "What will you have tonight, sir?"

MY ANSWER: "ICE WATER, PLEASE."

(**Sidenote:** I have been looking for the culprit who put that condom on my penis for sixteen years, and I have yet to find him. You have a lot of explaining to do when I do find you. You can run, but you cannot hide.)

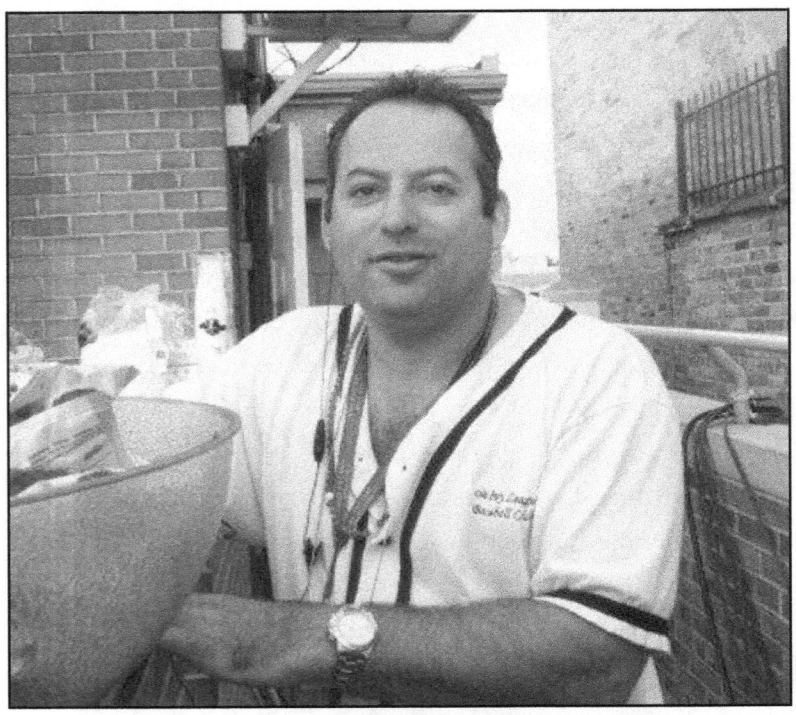

Max Waisvisz is one of the owners of Gold Coast Tickets in Chicago. Here is Max on his rooftop across the street from Wrigley Field.

MY BACKGROUND: THE EARLY YEARS

April 1963 to September 1981

MY NAME IS Eddie Arana, short for Edward Anthony Arana. I was born on April 9, 1963, in San Francisco, California. My parents, Carlos and Aida Arana, both of Peruvian descent, moved me and my older sister by one year, Virginia, to Chicago, Illinois, within six months of my birth. So, I consider myself a Chicagoan and a 100-percent Peruvian.

We grew up very middle class on the North Side of Chicago, living in three North Side Chicago neighborhoods from when I was six months old through to my twenties—Rogers Park, Edgewater, and finally Jefferson Park. My childhood was absolutely fabulous. I grew up in an extremely loving household. My dad worked as a sales promotion manager at Binks Manufacturing Co. in Franklin Park, Illinois. I had no idea what a sales promotion manager did when I was young, but he did wear a suit every day and we knew not to bother him when he came home from work every night. My mom stayed home and took care of me and my older sister.

My mom always claimed that she graduated from the University of Southern Mississippi. However, upon further review, I discovered that she had never even been to the state of Mississippi. I knew what she was doing—she was trying to instill in us the idea that college was important and that we needed to pursue a higher education after high school.

One of my earliest memories involving my mom was when I was six or seven years old, when we were living in Rogers Park. My mom and I would play catch with a baseball. She had a pretty good arm for a middle-aged Peruvian woman. I wore a baseball mitt while she did not. Anytime any of the neighborhood kids came around, I would run and hide from them. I didn't want any of the kids seeing that I was playing with my mom—I was ashamed. Maybe I wanted to be known as an independent person or a "tough guy."

My dad was the most popular person I knew growing up. His given name was Carlos, but everyone called him Ed or Eddie. He had many friends, and my parents would host countless parties at our house. Everyone loved my dad. His sense of humor was second to none. He treated everyone with respect, especially my mom. He would hold her hand as they walked down the street—always.

Every night when my dad came home from work, my mom would make him a steak, her famous white rice with corn in it, and a salad. My dad liked his steak rare. He always told my mom to "error rare." He meant that once a piece of meat has been overcooked, there is nothing that can be done to save that meat—it is ruined. However, if you undercook a piece of meat, it can be fixed by cooking it some more. Hence, if you have to make an "error" cooking meat, make sure the error is on the rare side.

One day, when I was twelve years old, my mom was making my dad his lunch—a bowl of soup along with a steak sandwich. Before she brought out the soup, I emptied a full bottle of Tabasco hot sauce into his bowl in the kitchen. I thought it would be hilarious to see his reaction when he started to eat his "spicy" soup. My mom begged me not to do it, but I convinced her that it would be okay. When he started to eat it, he took about four or five spoonsful of the soup and didn't seem fazed at all. I was thinking to myself, How is this possible? There is enough Tabasco in that bowl of soup to kill a lesser man. After a few more spoonsful, my dad looked up at me and smiled and said, "Soup's got a little bite to it, doesn't it Eddie?" This was the kind of relationship I had with my Dad. He was my idol.

I attended St. Gregory Grammar School from fifth through eighth grade (1975 to 1978). It was during these years that I was first introduced to alcohol. Some of the guys from the neighborhood began to experiment with beer. I was fascinated by this. I didn't do anything about it, however, but I did think it was extremely interesting. My parents had taught me at a very early age that drinking was an adult thing and that I should not try it until I was much older.

I absolutely despised it when my either of my parents drank, which was not very often. I especially hated whenever my mom drank. I hated the change of personality, which I could instantly detect. I could also tell when my dad drank, even if he had had only one drink. His behavior changed, and I did not like that at all. Why would someone put something in their body in order to change who they really are? I vowed never to drink alcohol because I hated to see how my parents acted under the influence. In hindsight, I should have listened to my own advice.

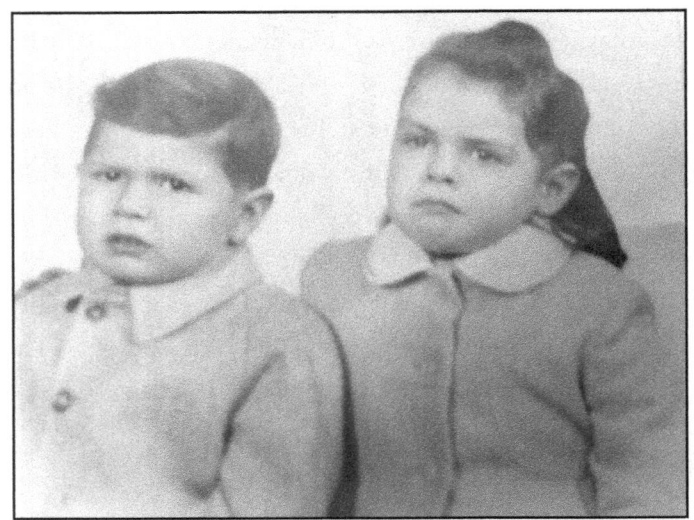

My sister, Virginia, and me looking very happy in Chicago.

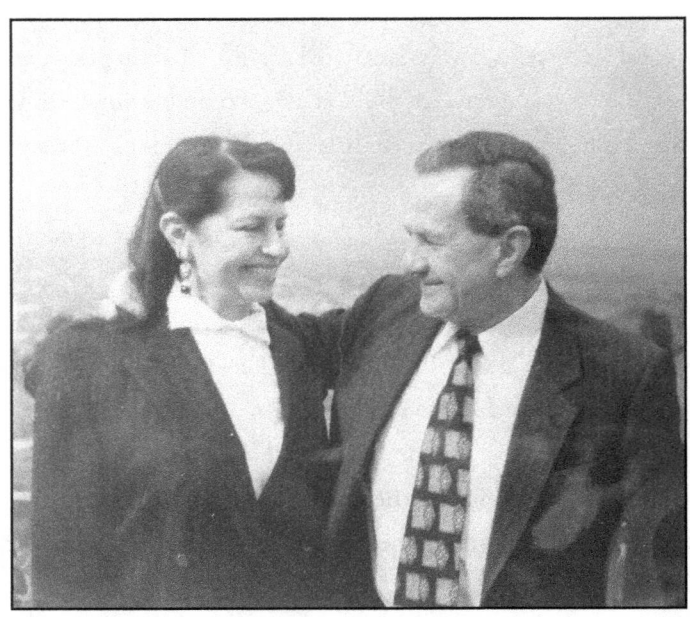

Mom and Dad staring into each other's eyes.

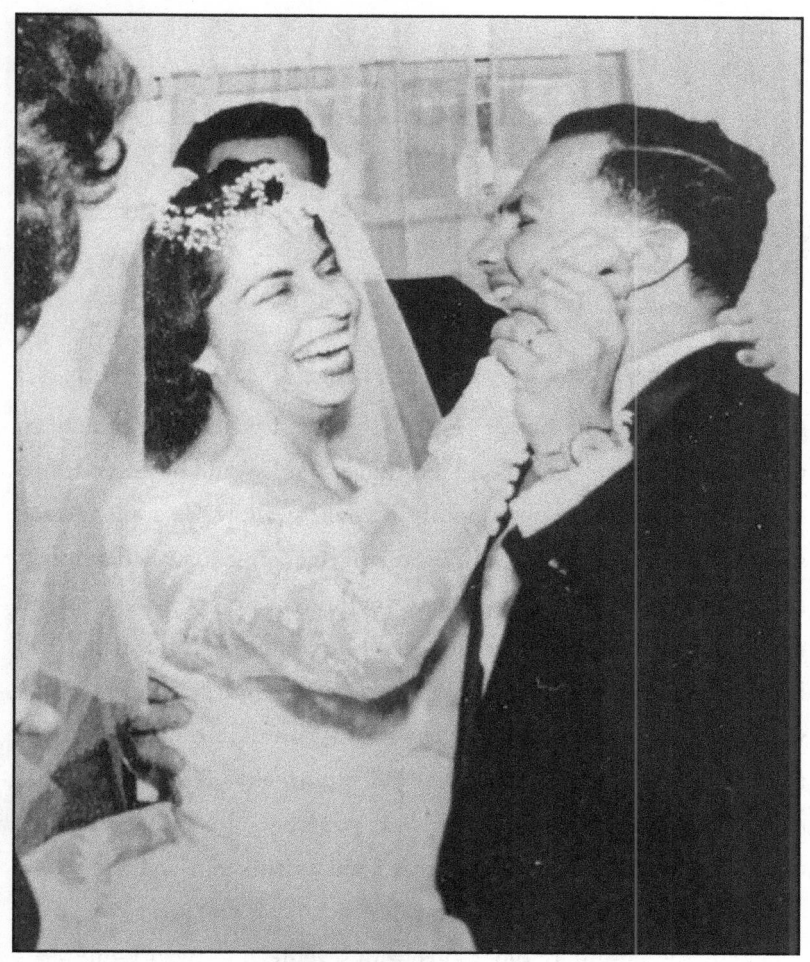

Mom and Dad dancing on their wedding day.

TEEN THOUGHTS

June 1976

AT THIRTEEN YEARS old, I belonged to a teen club in the Edgewater neighborhood on the North Side of Chicago. I walked the mile or so to this club from my house on Hermitage, and I would have about two ounces of apple juice in my mouth. I would swallow the apple juice as soon as I would get to the club. I thought that apple juice had a similar smell to alcohol—beer, to be exact. My thought process was so fucked up: I actually wanted my friends at the teen club to think that I had been drinking, even though I was too scared to actually drink. Just writing this is so embarrassing. Why the fuck would a thirteen-year-old think like that? I know why. That kid was an alcoholic in training. I equated alcohol with popularity and "coolness." I wanted people to think that I was "cool," too, and that I was a drinker.

Please talk to me, I wished. I am just as cool as you are.

There was a group of older kids from seventeen to twenty-one years old who gathered at the corner of Thorndale Avenue and Hermitage Avenue every night in the summer. They would be drinking beer, usually Old Style. They would play loud music through their Jensen tri-axle car speakers, and there would always be pretty girls around them——girls I could never even talk to. It seemed all of the girls wanted to be with the guys who were drinking. Whenever those guys drank beer, they became popular. I worshipped them. They were legends in my mind. They were who I aspired to be.

Here was my train of thought:

> *If I drink, I would be cool.*
> *If I drink, I could have a car and play loud music.*
> *If I drink, I could be talking to pretty girls.*

I would have loved to join them, but my parents had ingrained in me that drinking was bad for me. At that point in my life, I didn't know anything about social status or money—or what money could buy. I just wanted to be as cool as those guys.

In order to fully fit in with them, I thought that I had to drink—a lot. And wow, did I succeed.

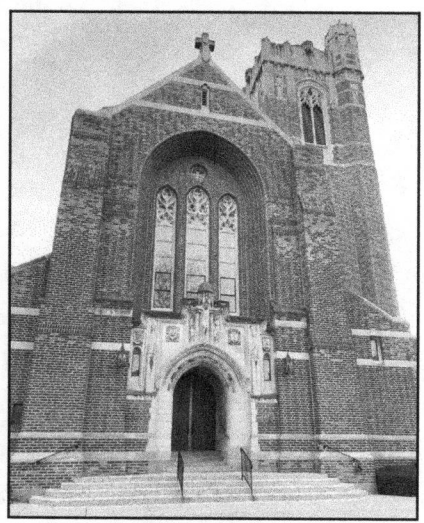

St. Gregory Church, located near the teen club
that I regularly walked to as a teenager.

GORDON TECH HIGH SCHOOL

September 1978 to June 1981

I WENT TO Gordon Tech High School (GT) on the corner of Addison Street and California Avenue in Chicago. I will always be a Gordon Tech Ram. I was in many honors classes at GT and I graduated ranked number one in the business program in 1981. (I have no idea why, but that was very difficult for me to write. I think this is the first time that I have actually acknowledged receiving that number-one ranking. With the friends I had at the time, I suppose it was not "cool" to be "smart.")

I was an honor student all four years of my high school career. My parents had instilled in me the importance of getting good grades in order to go to college. But I could not let on to my friends that I was smart. I didn't want anyone to know. Cool guys weren't smart. I bought two separate sets of school books starting my sophomore year. I left one set of books at school and one set of books at home. I did this to give the appearance that I never brought my books home to study. I would just ride the bus home with my friends and pretend that I didn't really give a shit about school, when, in actuality, I would be rushing home in order to finish my homework before dinner.

On one particular morning, as my friends and I were sitting in the GT cafeteria having our usual donuts and chocolate milk, a classmate of mine came over to our table and handed me an application for the National Honor Society (NHS), which was the nation's premier organization established to recognize outstanding high school students. He told me to fill out the application because it was due at the end of the week and being part of the NHS would help me get into college. My friend Danny McCarthy, who was six-foot-one and weighed about 285 pounds (in high school), snatched the application from my hand and tore it up right in front of everyone. He announced to the whole table:

"Fuck that. You don't need that honors shit."

I was so angry with him that I instinctively slapped him hard across the side of his head. I did not say a word, and he knew I was pissed. He stared back at me, and I knew what was coming next—either a punch in the face or a retaliatory slap. I felt like time stood still as we stared at each other for what seemed like an eternity. Then he just sat down and shook his finger at me, saying:

"You are fucking lucky I like you, or you would be in a hospital right now."

The point of the story is that intelligence and trying to improve oneself through education was not a driving force in the life I spent with the group of guys I hung out with. They were more focused on loyalty to the group and having a good time. I had to prove myself socially more than I had to prove myself intellectually.

I never went to a dance in high school, and I never went to the senior prom that most of my friends attended. I was too afraid to ask a girl to prom for fear that I would be rejected. Though I wasn't an outcast, I was just very nervous around women and I did not have one ounce of confidence.

Somehow, I managed to avoid drinking during the first couple of years of my high school career. I was very proud of the fact that I received straight A's throughout high school at Gordon Tech. However, I only told a few people about it. I didn't want to be known as the "smart guy."

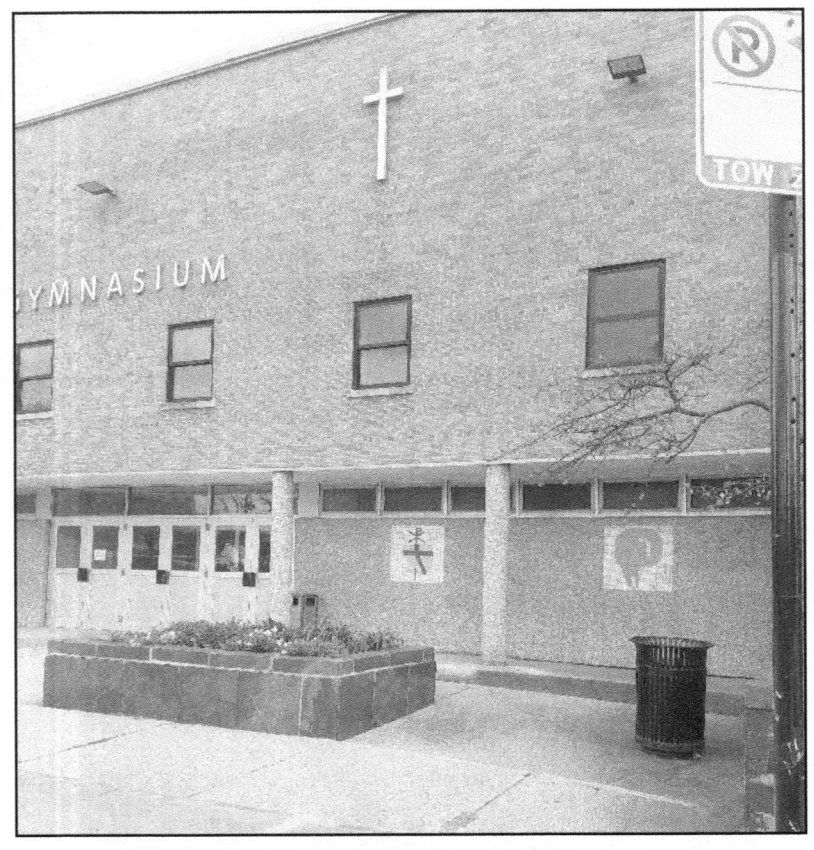

Gordon Tech High School, home of the Rams!
GT was located on the corner of Addison and California in Chicago.

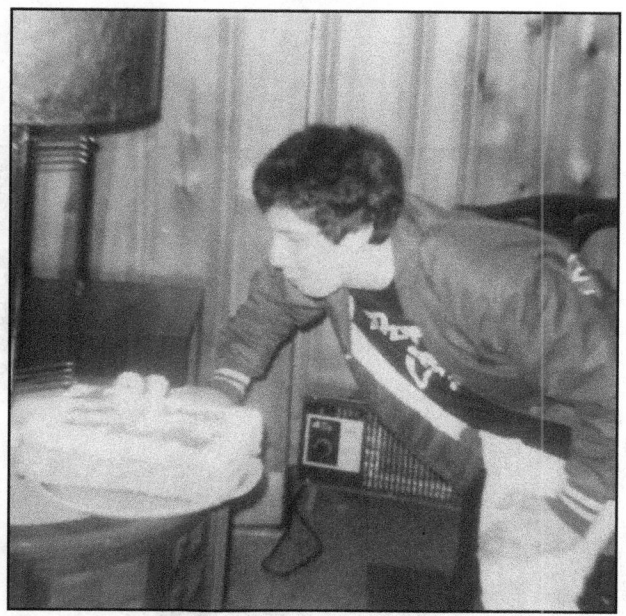

Blowing out the candles on my eighteenth birthday

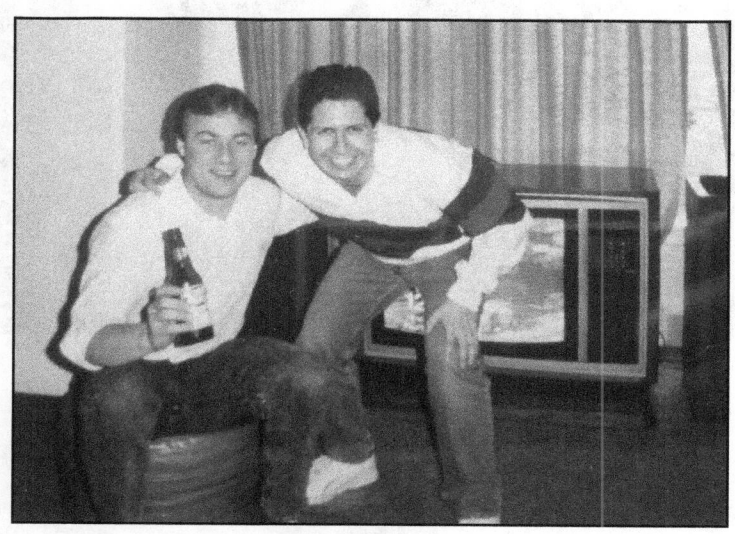

Mike Milazzo—one of my best friends—getting ready for another night out.

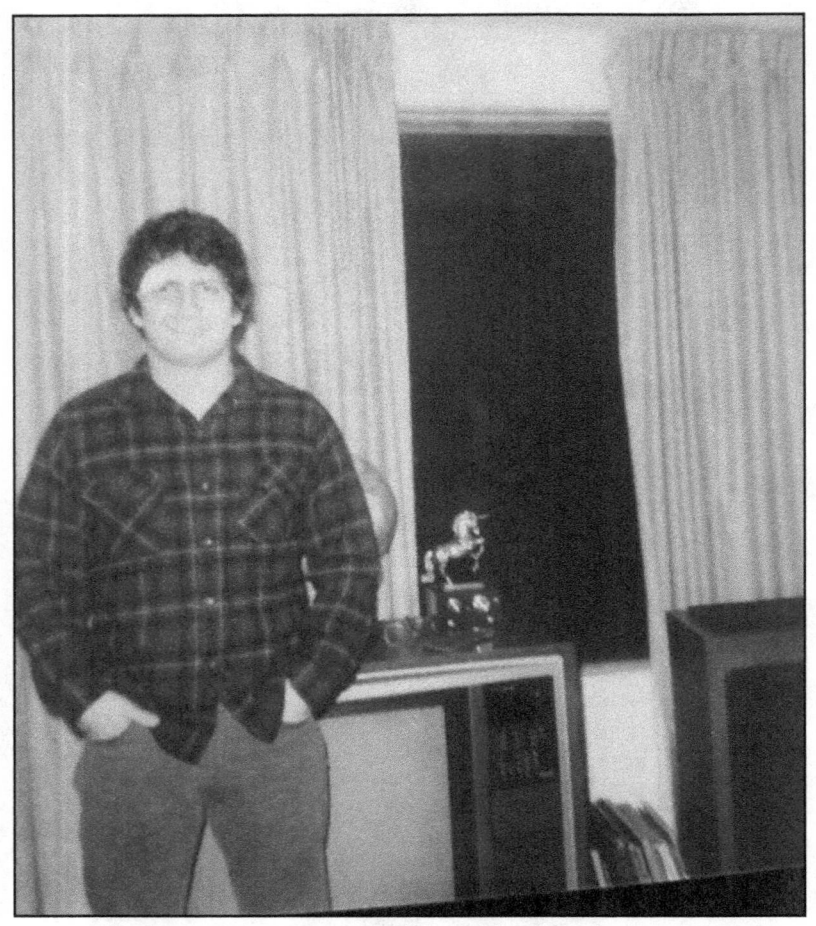

Here I am, smiling after a minor eye injury after a fight.

MY FIRST DRINK

August 9, 1979

THE FIRST TIME I ever drank alcohol was on August 9, 1979. I was sixteen years old. I was in the basement of my parent's house on Hermitage Avenue by myself. My dad had a large bottle of Chivas Regal (Scotch whiskey), which was in a pendulum-like wooden cradle that made it easier to pour because the bottle was so heavy. My mom was going to take me and my sister to ChicagoFest, an outdoor music festival in Navy Pier, to see the Scorpions perform live in concert that evening.

I was a huge fan of the Scorpions, and I was super excited about going to my first concert. Most of my friends had already been experimenting with alcohol by this time, and I had somehow resisted the temptation because, in my mind, I knew it was wrong to drink before you were twenty-one years old. But something must have snapped inside my mind because on this particular day, I felt different. I took a shot glass and poured one drink into it because I wanted to feel good and prepare myself for the Scorpions. The whiskey had a horrible taste. How could anyone enjoy this? And I didn't feel anything. So, I took another shot. The same thing happened. It had a horrible taste, and I did not feel a thing. So, I took a third shot, and a fourth, and a fifth, and a sixth, and a seventh . . .

The next thing I remember was waking up in my bed with the room spinning. My immediate reaction was not that I had done something terrible and that I would never do it again; instead, I was pissed off that I had missed the concert. Before we could leave, my mom had caught me acting all goofy, and we did not make it to ChicagoFest that night. I knew my mom was mad at me, and I was scared. I wish I could have truly appreciated the pain that I know my mom felt when she saw me drunk for the first time. I now know what that pain feels like as a parent. But at the time, I did not care. When I woke up that night, I was still very scared, but I was also excited that I had discovered that drinking could make me feel this way.

I had a feeling in my head—the buzz—that I thought was heavenly. I wanted to feel like this again. I wanted to feel like this every day of my life. It was the best feeling in the world. This was the feeling that I would eventually chase my entire drinking career. I also felt that it was very interesting that I chose to drink for the first time by myself. Maybe I didn't want anyone around me because I knew in my heart of hearts that it was not the right thing to do. Maybe I didn't want anyone to see that I was doing a bad thing. But my curiosity got the best of me. It was a situation that was bound to happen. I have always wondered if I would have gotten that drunk if my first drink had been with my group of friends.

The overwhelming feeling I had that day was guilt. However, the buzz trumped the guilt—that day and every day that followed.

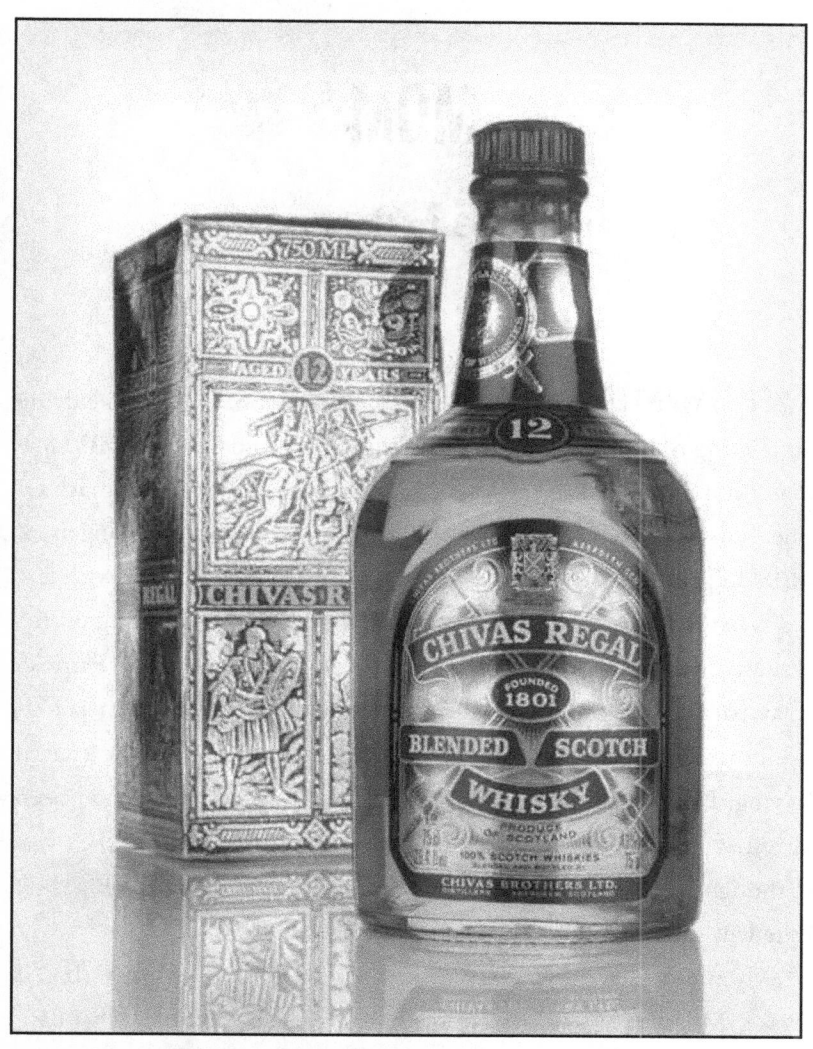

A bottle similar to the one that I poured my very first drink out of.

MOM

April 1963 to the Present

I *NEVER* WANTED to lose the feeling of my first buzz. It was like dying and going to heaven. You can drink something and feel like this? How had I not discovered this before? My Mom took the "soft" approach on me. That first night, she gave me a stern lecture on the dangers of drinking and told me never to do it again. I had gotten away with it.

When I was seventeen years old, I was arrested for drinking on the subway with my good friend, Pete Eberle, on my way to the St. Patrick's Day parade in Downtown Chicago. I was doing push-ups in jail—I was that drunk. When my mom found out about this, she started crying. I could see the disappointment in her eyes. Her son had been arrested. Again, I was lectured and "grounded" for a week. At the time, I thought, hey, we all have to take a punishment, right? No big deal. She will get over it.

My mom knew that every time I would go out with my friends Piske, Milazzo, Marco, or Nino, there would be trouble. This happened in my late teens and into my twenties. Every parent out there who sees their kids going out on a weekend night knows exactly what I'm talking about. Again, I did not care what my mom thought or said to me. In retrospect, the parents of Piske, Milazzo, Marco, and Nino should have been worried about their sons going out with *me*. I was the bad crowd they should have avoided.

I would constantly see the pain and worry in my mom's face, and I really didn't care. She would wait up for me until all hours of the night just to make sure that I came home alive. I would barely give my mom a hello when I would eventually get home and just pass out in my room. All she wanted to do was talk to me and make sure I was safe. All she wanted was to have some normal time with her son whom she loved so much.

When I got married, we had been doing some construction to our house, so we moved in to my parents' house for about six months. It was a glorious time. My mom would cook every night for myself, my wife, and the kids. And we had free babysitting, so I would go out with my friends all the time. My mom would be so worried and would lecture me:

"Te vas a perder todo!" ("You are going to lose everything!") My reaction? I laughed in her face. I thought that she had no clue about young people. Didn't she know we were invincible? Wasn't she aware that young people could get away with anything and not face any consequences? Had she not gotten that memo?

One night during our stay at my parents' house, I was involved in a major accident on the Kennedy Expressway. I fell asleep at the wheel while I was drunk at 3 a.m. Luckily, I walked away from the accident, and literally walked home to my parent's house. I had to explain to my mom what had happened. I could tell she was devastated. I didn't understand. I was fine. I was not hurt. What's the big fucking deal?

Fast forward to 2004, I was involved in another major car accident that would change my life and lead me on the path toward sobriety. It was the last straw. I got charged with a DUI. It led to my divorce. And

I did lose everything—I lost my family and the ability to see my kids. Drinking was the main cause of the devastation that I left behind in my wake, and I was too fucking stupid to realize it when I was in the middle of it.

I hope that the kids who read this book realize what they are doing to their parents. I'll bet 99 out of 100 will laugh at this. I don't care about the 99. I care about the one whom I can help.

I should have listened to you, Mom. You were right. I'm sorry.

I am not laughing anymore.

My mom passed away peacefully during the writing of this book on February 1, 2020. My mom was so worried about my drinking over the years, and I am so happy that for the last fifteen years of her life, I was sober. I owed her at least that much. She loved sober Eddie. We never discussed my drinking during those fifteen years, but I knew that she knew that I was finally "safe."

One of my last "sobriety hurdles" was the passing of one of my parents. Would this lead me to drink? One of my biggest fears in life was realized. I am proud to let everyone know that I did not drink. I came very close the night before she passed away, but a little voice in the back of my head told me not to.

Thank you, Mom. I will always love you.

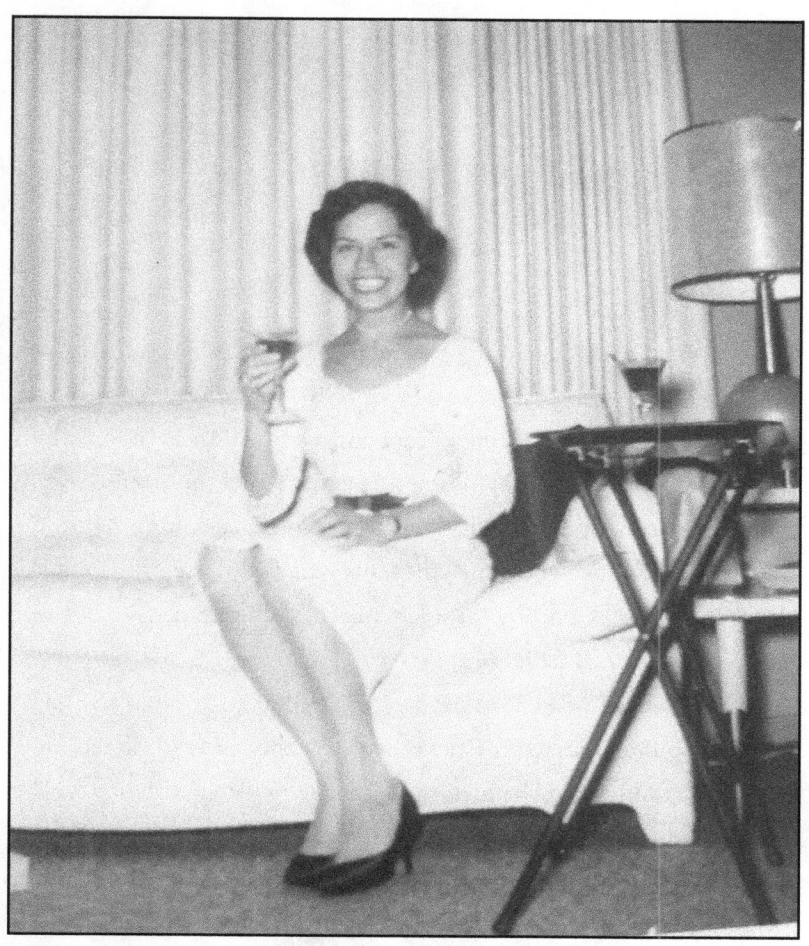

My Mom—the living saint—Aida Arana.

DAD

April 1963 to the Present

MY DAD WAS small in stature, but he was a giant to me. When I was growing up, he worked six days a week. He would always come home from work with a big smile on his face and a steak dinner ready for him to devour—prepared by my mom. After his dinner, he would love to sit on the couch and watch TV with me, mostly sporting events. We loved all of the Chicago teams—the Cubs, the Bears, the Bulls, and the Blackhawks. Yes, I purposefully left off the White Sox. We did not consider them a real Chicago sports team.

My dad would often take me to Wrigley Field to watch the Cubs play. He would approach the ticket window about ten to fifteen minutes before the start of the game and ask the ticket attendant what he had available for the day. My dad would then slip the guy some extra money, and we would always end up with the best seats in the house. It was like heaven for me to be at a Cubs game with my dad; I could not imagine a better afternoon. My dad never drank at the game—not one time. I was so proud to be there in those great seats watching my favorite team.

My dad was my biggest fan. Whenever his friends came over to visit, he would always call me from my room and have me greet his friends and talk to them. He would brag about how well I was doing at school or how good I was at sports. My dad was not the disciplinarian in our house—it was definitely my mom. My dad would always give me a knowing smile of reassurance whenever I was in trouble. He never wanted me to feel bad about anything. I loved that about him.

My dad loved to drink when he had parties at our house. Those parties would last until all hours of the night. I had recollections of loud Peruvian music and my dad playing the maracas. He was a master at playing those maracas. I never went downstairs when those parties were going on. I hated seeing my parents while they were drinking; it made me sick to my stomach.

One night, my parents came home from a holiday party, and my dad had driven them home. The next morning, my dad noticed that he had left the driver-side door of his car wide open. He was so scared and appalled that he had been drinking and driving in that fashion that he said he would stop drinking. He was forty-one years old at the time, and I was thirteen. He never drank in front of me again. He never went to any AA meetings or anything like that, either. He just stopped. I was so grateful. I, too, stopped drinking at forty-one years of age—like father, like son.

My dad also passed away during the writing of this book on July 6, 2020. This was my final drinking hurdle. Again, my lifelong fear had always been one of my parents dying. Now, they were both gone. This was the one time when I would have had a perfectly legitimate excuse to get drunk just one final time. No one would ever know. My hero was gone, and I felt so alone. I knew exactly where I would go to drink—Here's Cheers Lounge on Oakton Street in Niles, Illinois. And I knew exactly what I was going to order—Glenlivet, neat.

I went to Cheers the night my dad passed away. The bartender asked me what I would like to drink. It was so hot that day—102 degrees with high humidity. My answer:

"Ice water, please."

Thanks, Dad. You taught me well.

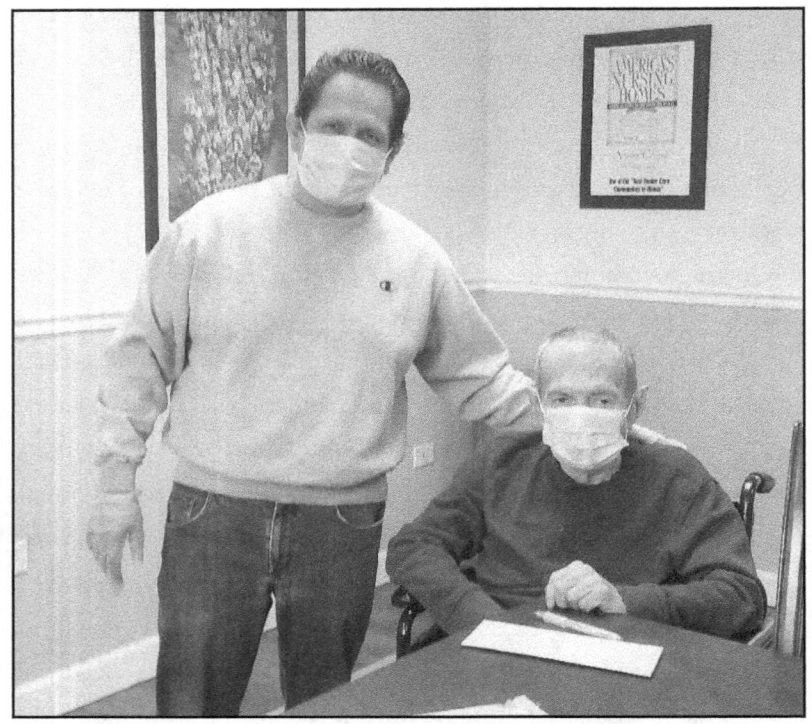

My Dad and I at Norwood Crossings Nursing Home.
This was the last time I saw my Dad before he passed away

RIDES HOME WITH ANIMALS

January 1981 to December 1990

MY DRINKING DURING my teenage years could be considered binge drinking. I just drank in order to get as drunk as I could to duplicate that first buzz I had attained in my parents' basement. When I got super drunk and had no way to get home, I would call my parents to pick me up. They would come at all hours of the night in their car armed with stuffed animals and full meals while I was falling down drunk.

I would say this happened about two hundred times in about ten years—from when I was about eighteen to twenty-eight years old. Typically, when I went out drinking with my friends, I would either get a ride home from a friend, walk, or take a cab, bus, or train. I hardly ever drove when I drank. (I believe I've only ever driven about ten times in total when I was drinking, and of those ten times, I was involved in four accidents—three of them major. So, I'd always made it a rule not to drink and drive. As we used to say in the old neighborhood: "I might be dumb, but I ain't stupid.") However, when I was done drinking, it was always very late, usually past 3 a.m. or so. I would outlast the person who had driven me there and the buses or trains, which would no longer be running. My only way home was to either walk or call my parents. Uber was not an option back in the old days.

My parents would come to pick me up in their car wherever I was. I would be sprawled out on a bus bench or just sitting on a sidewalk or still drinking inside a late-night tavern. My mom would get out of the car and let me sit in the front, taking her spot in the back of the car. She was extremely old-school Peruvian in that way. My dad always drove with a huge smile on his face. Looking back on it, that smile must have been a smile of relief when he saw that I was still alive.

Let's keep in mind that my mom was a living saint. I do not believe she had ever done anything wrong in her life, and, under questioning, I believe she would testify that she didn't believe I had ever done anything wrong, either. She would be carrying a Curious George stuffed animal (or other similar stuffed monkey toy—there were many of them in the house so she had plenty to choose from) that she would hand to me. I would sit the monkey on my lap sort of like a little baby. She would also have a large plate of freshly cooked T-bone or rib eye steak (prepared medium-rare), along with a large portion of her award-winning white rice with corn mixed in. She would also have a smaller plate of salad with thinly sliced tomatoes, drizzled with either Thousand island or Italian dressing. Also, she would have apple juice, grape juice, or Hawaiian Punch (Fruit Juicy Red) ready in a juice box. One thing I do not remember being there was salt or pepper. That would have been a nice touch. I would enjoy this meal on my way home in the car in the front seat. You can imagine me trying to cut the steak with a knife and fork and eating a gourmet meal while my dad drove us home—and I would just be talking gibberish and nonsense the entire ride. The food was always delicious—perfectly prepared.

What I wasn't aware of at the time, while I enjoyed my steak in the front seat after a night out of drinking, was what my parents had to do behind the scenes. My parents would be woken up from a deep sleep at 3 a.m. and get ready to pick me up. My mom would have to prepare a full meal in the early hours of the morning—and she would only have about ten or fifteen minutes to prepare it. I really thought this was a perfectly normal thing for parents to do. How fucked up is that? My parents did this for me at least two hundred more times in my life even after I put them through hell. This is what is referred to as "unconditional love." This love believes that your child can do no wrong. This love believes that food will make everything okay. This love believes that this is the last time you ever have to pick up your child looking and acting like a man possessed.

I cannot believe I put those poor people through all of that. If I knew the damage that I caused and the pain and suffering I put on my parents, I would never have done what I did . . . wait a minute. I was a fucking alcoholic—of course I would have done it over and over and over again! It is amazing how much control alcohol has over your decision making, especially at a young age. My parents meant the world to me, and I had zero to little respect for them. Now, they are my heroes. Unconditional love.

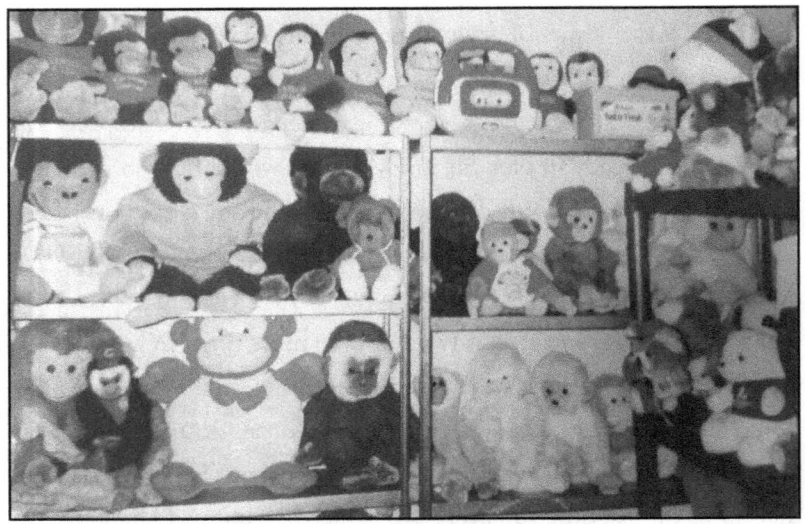

Here is just a sampling of the collection of
monkeys at my mom's house on Argyle Street.

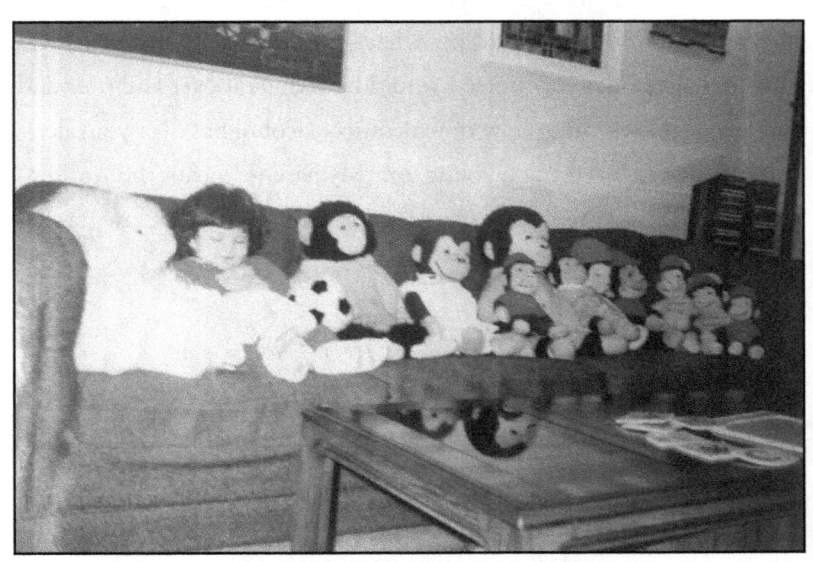

My daughter Sarah enjoying some quiet time with my monkeys.

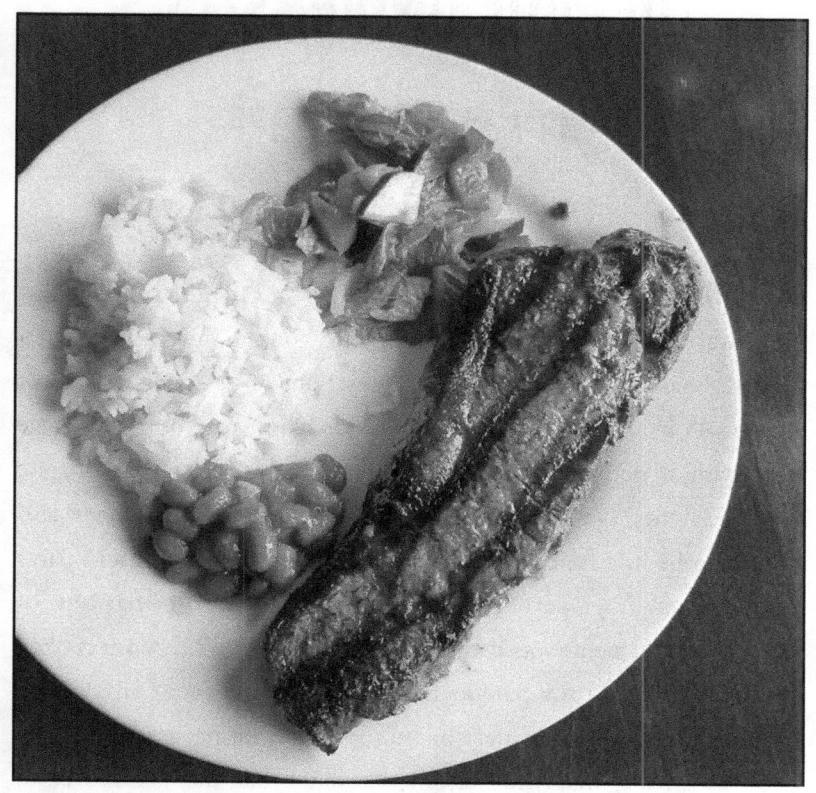

Picture of steak and rice (prepared by myself)—very similar to the
kind of meal my mom would have ready for me in the car after
my parents picked me up from my drunk nights out.

DEPAUL UNIVERSITY

August 1981 to June 1985

I ATTENDED DEPAUL University in Chicago and majored in accounting. I was a pretty smart guy. I could have gone to any college that I wanted. I had gotten straight A's in high school, and my goal was to get straight A's in college. Many of my friends who were going to college were dying to go far away to school. They went to various out-of-state schools so they could get the whole "college experience"; they also wanted to be in a fraternity and live in a dorm and go out and party every night at "toga parties." I had very little interest in that type of scenario. My homelife was already so great in my eyes. My mom cooked the best meals, and my parents never bothered me about anything. I had a feeling that my parents wanted me to stay home, as well.

My sister, Virginia, who was one year older than me, had moved to San Francisco when I was a senior at DePaul. Virginia had just graduated from Northwestern University. She had gone to the Medill School of Journalism, which was one of the most prestigious journalism schools in the country. She would write papers for her journalism classes that I could not understand even if my life depended on it. Virginia was the smartest person I knew. I felt mentally inferior to her. She was my best friend. I cried like a baby the day she left to go to the airport. I felt like she had abandoned me. She absolutely despised my drinking. She would lecture me about it every time she caught me drunk, and I never wanted to hear about it from her—especially her.

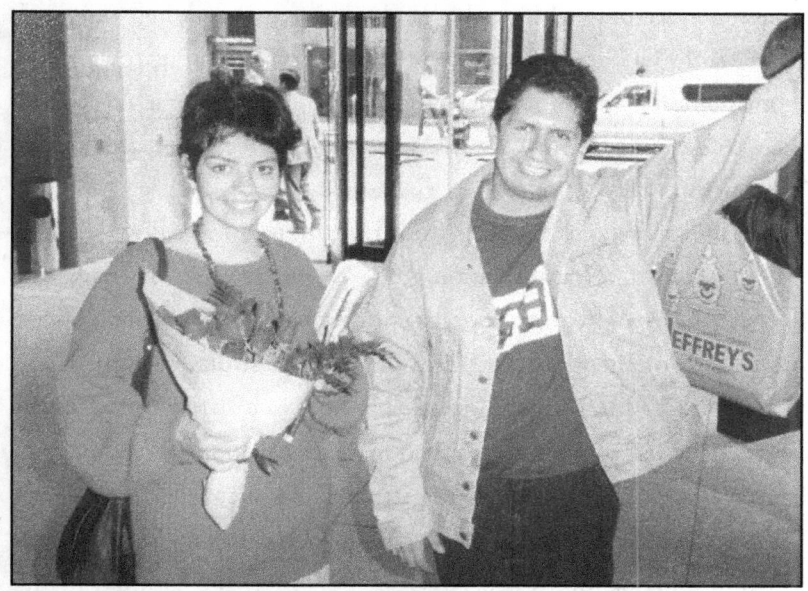

My sister, Virginia, and I in San Francisco during a weekend visit.

Perhaps part of the reason I wanted to stay in Chicago also had to do with my core group of drinking friends. These friends included Jimmy Piske, Yaki Halter, Nino Speciale, Mike Milazzo, and Marco Simonetti. I didn't want to "leave them behind," so to speak. These friends did not go to college; they went right to work after high school. I really admired that. I had a very blue-collar work ethic with a white-collar education, one might say.

DePaul was just an extension of high school, for me. I also bought two different sets of school books in college—one set for home and the other set for school. Again, I did not want people to know that I was smart. The accounting program was a very difficult one, so I really had to dedicate myself to studying during the week. I was extremely disciplined in my study habits. Sunday nights through Thursday nights were spent at home with my books doing intense studying sessions. I never went to a library. I had the perfect atmosphere in my own room in my home. My parents were never loud. You could hear a pin drop in their house. And any meal I wanted would be perfectly prepared by my mom within thirty minutes.

My life goal was to graduate from DePaul, pass the CPA (Certified Public Accountant) examination, get a decent job, get married, and live happily ever after. As I look back on things, I never really mapped out those aforementioned goals in any type of structured way. I just knew that I had to get good grades in school in order to be successful in life. This was something that had been taught to me by my parents at a very early age. I succeeded in getting all A's in college.

I mentioned that Sunday nights through Thursday nights were dedicated to studying for my college classes. So, Friday and Saturday nights were spent "studying" for my drinking life. I studied equally as hard for that part of my life, as well. I wanted to get "straight A's" in drinking so I could impress my friends.

During my senior year at DePaul, I had an interview at Ernst & Whinney, which at the time was a top accounting firm in Chicago. I had gone out drinking the night before the interview and had gotten into a fight, which sent me to the hospital where I received three stitches over my left eye. I walked into the interview with a large white bandage over my eye. The interviewer asked me what I knew about the company. My response was, "Well, I know you are growing." Then there were ten seconds of awkward silence as the interviewer waited for a little more from me in terms of a response—which he never got.

I did not get the job. The interviewer must have taken one look at me and my bandage and crossed me off of the list.

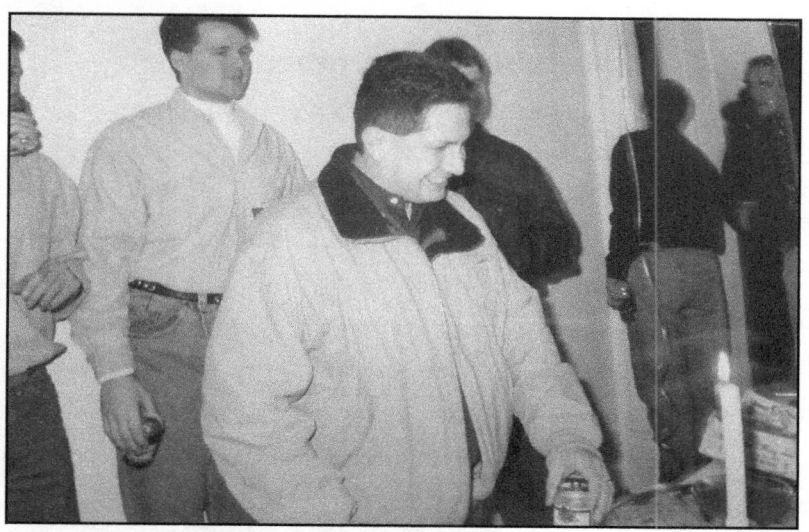

Surprise, Eddie! Happy Birthday! My parents threw me a surprise party; I was around twenty years old.

EARLY DRINKING PATTERNS

June 1980 to December 1990

I NEVER LIKED the taste of alcohol. As a matter of fact, I hated it. I would marvel at the people who would say:

"I wish I had a nice cold beer right now."

In my mind, a "nice cold beer" is the last thing I would want to quench my thirst. I would prefer a Mott's apple juice or a Welch's grape juice or a Hawaiian Punch Fruit Juicy Red. Even water would be a much more logical choice for me. The taste of beer, especially the aftertaste, was abhorrent to me. I still feel that way to this day.

My fascination with alcohol was the effect that it had on me, especially at a young age. After my experimentation with Chivas Regal (my first drinking experience), I stuck with beer for the most part. I would drink so quickly because I hated the taste so much that I could not wait for the drink to be done with. I usually drank a twelve-ounce beer in about three or four gulps. Naturally, every beer following your first beer of the day or night gets easier and easier to drink.

I preferred less filling beers such as Miller Lite. Many of my friends drank Guinness, a dark stout beer from Ireland. I thought Guinness was the devil. I would rather have several dentist appointments than drink a Guinness. All that being said, if my friends and I were sitting in an Irish pub and the bartender asked me what I wanted to drink, I would announce:

"Guinness, please! What else would I drink?"

I did not want to be known as a "soft" drinker or a "pussy." Being an "accomplished" or "seasoned" drinker was a major deal to me. I wanted to learn about drinking and what was appropriate to drink and at what time and place it was appropriate to do so. Thankfully, when you are still young, you can stick with beer and an occasional shot of whiskey, and you will not be known as a drinking pariah.

My early drinking years consisted of many drinking episodes. The formula was always the same: I would start out drinking very fast and get very intoxicated. I would then proceed to do some very stupid and/or insensitive things. Then I would regret my actions. I knew they were wrong. However, they did give me the attention that I desired so badly. I chose the attention over morality.

Here are a few examples:

A group of friends and I went to see Led Zeppelin's concert movie *The Song Remains the Same* at midnight at the Nortown Theater on the North Side of Chicago. I woke up after the movie ended at 8 a.m. (the following day), laid out between two rows of seats at the theater. My head and hair were basically glued to the floor because of the popcorn butter that had apparently stuck to my head. I had urinated all over myself and

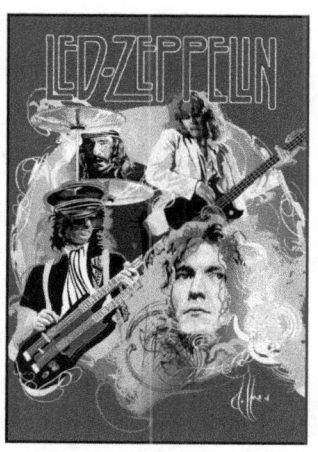

Led Zeppelin was my favorite band growing up.

had an empty bottle of Jack Daniel's and a bottle of blackberry brandy in my pocket.

Once, Jack "Yaki" Halter and I had gone out drinking on Christmas Eve night. This was during the Cabbage Patch Kids craze in the early eighties where these dolls were the hottest Christmas toys available. Yaki and I went back to his parents' house and decided to do snow angels on his front lawn at about three o'clock in the morning in a very loud and obnoxious way. Yaki's little sister, Sonja, had woken up during the commotion and went outside, wondering what was going on. I yelled over to her, "Hey Sonja, did you get your Cabbage Patch doll for Christmas yet?"

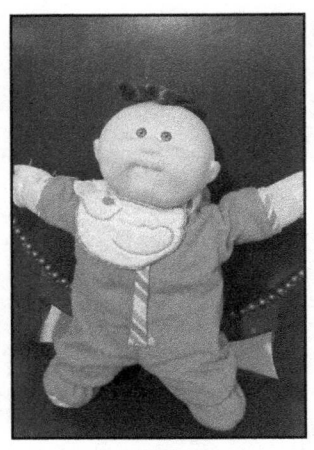

A Cabbage Patch Kid doll similar to the one Yaki's sister, Sonja, received for Christmas.

Apparently, I had forgotten that Santa Claus had not arrived at their house yet. Sonja started crying and yelling to her mother, "Mom! Eddie and Yaki ruined Christmas again!"

Another time, my Gordon Tech High School classmates and I had just gotten our junior class rings, which was a big deal at our school. My parents had paid $175 for my ring. A few of my friends had decided to go to the top of a hill at Warren Park on Western Avenue in Chicago. I had been drinking the entire afternoon. As a group, we decided to throw our rings from the hill on the count of three. It sounded like a great idea to me at the time. Apparently, I was the only one who threw my ring away on three. We looked for my ring for over two hours and never found it.

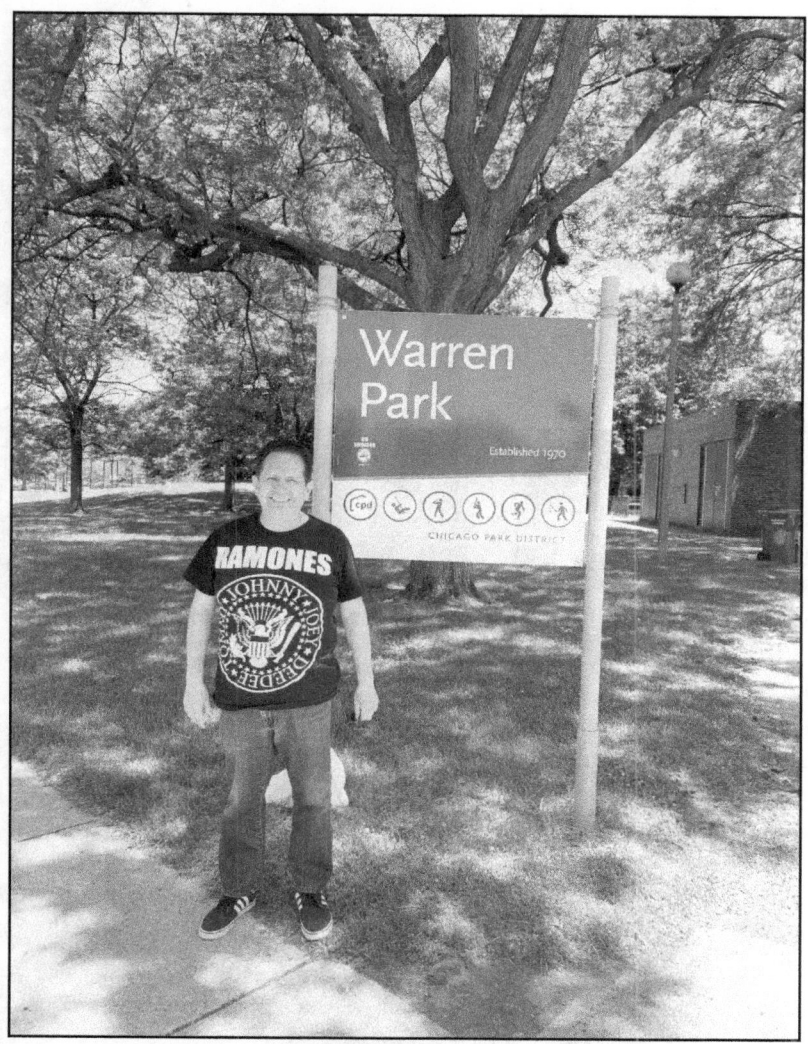

Back to the scene of the original crime at Warren Park
where I threw away my class ring.

Once, I accidentally spilled an entire sixteen-ounce beer on an Indian girl in the Wrigley Field bleachers on a hot afternoon at a Cubs game. She called the security guard over and complained that my group of friends and I were way overserved and that we needed to be kicked out. I knew the head of security at Wrigley Field, and he approved our staying in our seats as long as we behaved. Two innings after the spilling incident, I vomited all over the same Indian girl's hair. We were then escorted out of the ballpark.

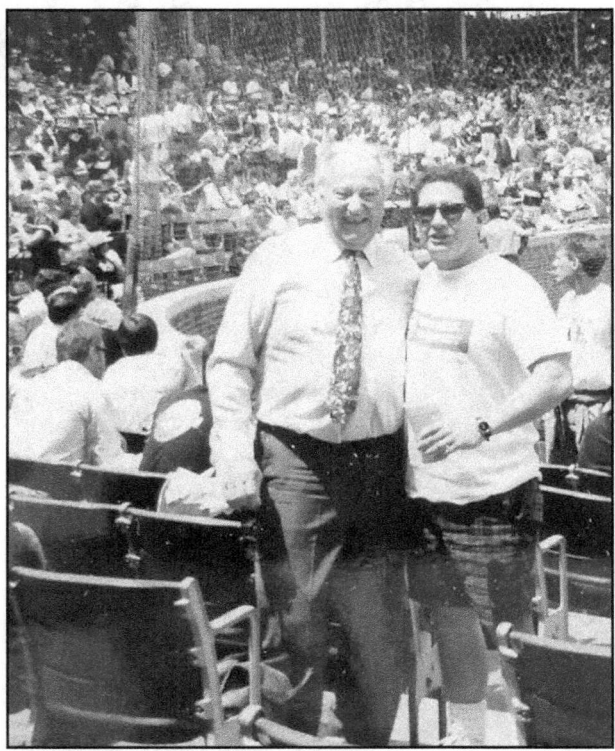

Taking a picture with Ray Meyer—famous DePaul University basketball legend—at Wrigley Field.

Another time, I received a letter in the mail that said I had finally passed my CPA examination. It had been my third attempt, and I was ecstatic. A group of us went to Barnaby's restaurant for pizza, breaded mushrooms, and beer. I did not tell anyone that I had passed the exam, even though it was a huge deal to me. Later that evening, we went to the Pumping Company on Broadway near Granville. I started to do shots of tequila and Jack Daniel's. When I went to the bathroom, I projectile vomited into the trough urinal. In order to impress my friend Jimmy Piske, I started to pick out the breaded mushrooms out of the vomit and ate them one by one.

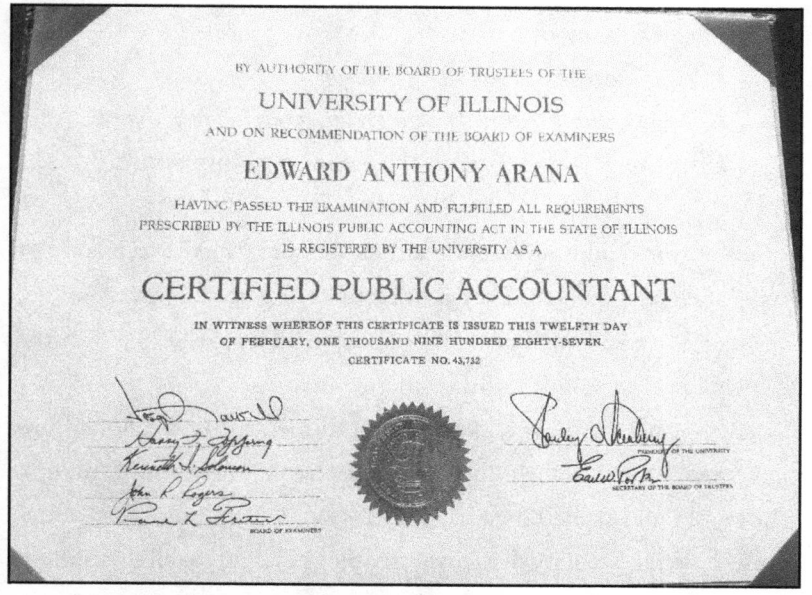

I am a CPA—shh! Don't tell anybody.

One time, my friends decided to throw me a "Find Eddie a Wife Party" at the Saratoga Bar & Grill located at Taylor Street and Loomis Street in Chicago's Little Italy neighborhood. I started drinking six hours before the event and do not even remember arriving at the party. There was a massive fight, where several of my friends received stitches, got arrested, and had to go to the hospital. The entire duration of the fight, which was outside of the bar, I was sleeping in one of the stalls of the men's bathroom.

The patterns in all of the stories above during my formative drinking years are very similar in nature:

> *I assembled my close friends.*
> *I drank quickly and got out of control.*
> *I did something either knowingly or unknowingly that I knew would get me, for lack of a better word, "recognition."*

In today's world, kids and young adults use social media to elevate or "hype" their social status. They post pictures of parties, or new clothes, or events they have attended. A lot of people do it for the "likes" or the "follows," or they simply do it for the "clout."

I did not have the convenience of social media. My alcohol adventures were chronicled through the telephone or word of mouth. Whenever I did something that I perceived as "hilarious" or "outrageous," I would quickly call as many people as I could to tell them about what I had done. Whether it was the truth or an exaggerated version, it didn't matter. I just wanted to get the story out there so I could be perceived as popular. I had found a way to "break through" socially. And it was a lot of fun. I loved getting drunk. I loved getting the attention that I had never gotten before. It was an amazing time in my life.

You may also notice a pattern in how much I swear in my drinking stories and my writing. (I apologize in advance if it is offensive to anyone.) My entire life, I grew up swearing (a lot) around my friends; however, I do not think I have ever used a swear word around my parents. Perhaps the swearing is a reflex that hearkens back to my drinking days. I would always be the loudest guy in the room. I wanted to be noticed, and swearing was one of the easiest ways to get noticed. And if you were swearing loudly, you would get noticed even faster. There is probably a psychiatrist out there somewhere salivating.

In many of my early drinking episodes, I encountered a very familiar scene that would happen again and again. It involved me looking into the mirror in the bathroom at whatever drinking establishment or house I happened to be drunk at. I would say to myself:

"What the fuck are you doing? You are ruining your life. You have to stop."

I recognized at a very early age, around eighteen, that this was not the right way to act or to live. I yelled at myself for disappointing my parents and myself. However, these bathroom remorse incidents would last about five or ten seconds. Immediately afterward, I would just return to my drinking business.

The drinking would always win.

CHICAGO MERCANTILE EXCHANGE

January 1986

MY FIRST WHITE-COLLAR job was at the Chicago Mercantile Exchange (CME) on South Wacker Drive in Downtown Chicago. I was hired as a staff auditor making a whopping $19,000 a year. My first day of work was January 27, 1986, and if you know anything about Chicago sports, you know that was the Monday after the Chicago Bears won the Super Bowl. The parade, which was attended by approximately five hundred thousand people in Downtown Chicago, was on Tuesday, January 28, 1986. This was not good timing for a person who drank as much as I did.

I had gone out drinking (heavily) that Saturday night on January 25 until 5 a.m. Sunday morning. I was already celebrating the Bears winning the Super Bowl the night before the game was even played. Everyone in Chicago was so sure of this Bears team winning the big game, and I was no different.

I was sleeping on the floor of the living room during almost the entire Super Bowl. My dad was sitting in his spot on the couch intently watching every play of the game. He had sporadically tried to wake me up during Bears touchdowns and great defensive plays, but for the most part, I slept through arguably the best game in the history of Chicago sports. And I was the biggest sports fan I knew. My dad and I would watch every Chicago sports game on television religiously. So for me to fall asleep during a Super Bowl—with the Bears in it and poised to win—was simply unfathomable.

I was fucking hung over and sleeping during the Chicago Bears Super Bowl victory! I still cannot believe that happened. What was I thinking?

I made it to work that Monday morning, and by Tuesday afternoon, I had discovered "after work drinking." I was fascinated by it. Everyone did it. There would always be someone willing to go out and drink after work. I was in an office where there were people my age (I was twenty-one) looking to get loose. Holy shit. Had I struck gold?

There is a major difference between drinking with your buddies and drinking with colleagues. You do not want to show your drinking hand, so to speak, too early. I figured out who the "cool" people in the office were immediately. These "cool" people could be defined as those who liked to drink. They were the people I migrated toward. I didn't want anything to do with the conservative, "boring" people who didn't appear to ever let loose.

I quickly rose through the ranks to be one of the top drinkers in the office. I was the King of Fun, as my first boss, Bill Pauly, once told me. I organized lunches. I organized trips to Wrigley Field for Cubs games. I organized get-togethers after work at different restaurants and bars downtown. I organized meetups at street festivals in the city. I was the social butterfly of the office. If anyone wanted to get a drink after work, they stopped at my desk to find out what the plans were. I tried to get everyone involved in the mix. And the one key ingredient that all of these outings shared was—you guessed it—alcohol.

I knew I had a drinking problem way back then. I knew that I did not drink like everyone else. But I didn't want anyone knowing about it. At least, I didn't want anyone knowing the extent of my problem. I used to come into work super early in the morning to copy blank pieces of paper at the copy machine just to show the bosses that I was at work on time and not hung over. I didn't want anyone to know that my drinking affected me whatsoever. I dedicated and organized my entire work day just so I could go out later that day and drink with my work friends. I was a good worker, but it was for all the wrong reasons.

The early years at the CME were some of the greatest drinking years of my life. I discovered "professional drinking," a.k.a. "drinking while wearing a suit." Somehow if you are wearing a suit, it makes drinking more acceptable. But I still drank the same way. I drank as fast as I could so I could get drunk faster. As I have stated before, I hated the taste of alcohol; I just loved being fucked up. But it was so important for me not to let anyone in on my dirty little secret: once I started, I could not stop. I would slur when I drank. I was loud when I drank. I said really stupid shit when I drank. I embarrassed myself when I drank. I embarrassed the people I was with when I drank. I didn't care about anything when I drank. However, I managed to hide it somewhat with different maneuvers that I now see, years later.

I was also extremely generous when I drank. I loved to buy people drinks. If you are buying, people tend to put up with you a lot longer. Money rights a lot of wrongs. I was buying people drinks with money that I should have kept in a savings account. My advantage was that I lived at home with my parents and did not have a car payment, so whatever I earned was disposable income. I managed to dispose my income at various bars in Downtown Chicago.

I was funny when I drank. I was quick with my wit and pretty good at making people laugh. Whether it was physical comedy (such as doing somersaults in a restaurant) or telling dirty jokes, I was pretty fucking entertaining. I was learning how to be a drunk and how not to get caught.

That was probably my most valuable lesson at the CME.

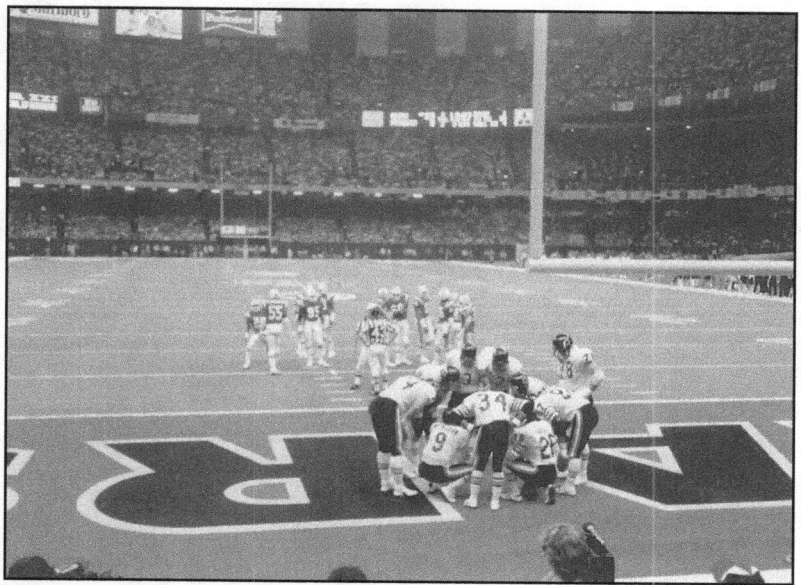

This was the greatest moment in Chicago sports history, which I slept through.

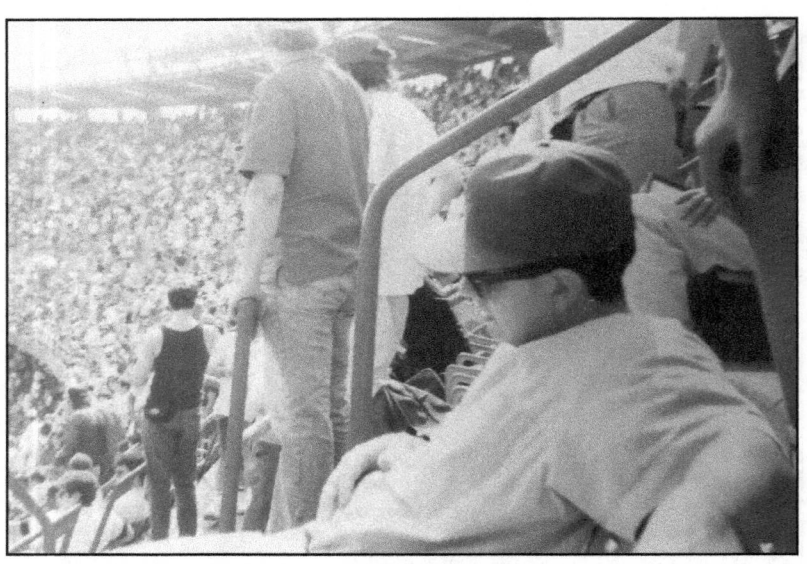

Falling asleep at a CME work outing. I am sure I was exhausted.

KING ARTHUR'S PUB AND JIMMY PISKE

November 1989

EVERYONE HAS THAT one friend you cannot say no to. Everything he suggests sounds like a great idea at the time. My friend was Jimmy Piske. Jimmy was the best drinking partner imaginable. When you are inebriated, he sounds like a genius. Everything he says makes perfect sense. Jimmy romanticized alcohol. He taught me about the subtle differences of alcohol and the different brand names and the tastes of different vodkas, tequilas, whiskeys, and beers; even though it all tasted the same to me—like shit. He once turned to me at a bar and uttered these words, "Drinking is fun!" I will never forget when he said that. I thought it was brilliant. Drinking *is* fun. Drinking can be the center of your universe, and why not have fun while you do it?

Jimmy worked at the Federal Reserve Bank in Downtown Chicago. He was a blond-haired, blue-eyed, very good-looking kid who grew up near Wrigley Field. In other words, he was everything I was not. He was over six feet tall—and I was short. He could talk to girls—and I could not. I looked up to Jimmy in many respects.

I introduced Jimmy to all of my friends at the Chicago Mercantile Exchange Audit Department, which was my first real job out of college. Jimmy was acutely aware of my drinking prowess and desire to constantly get drunk. Jimmy and I would go out every Friday after work, and I would blow most of my biweekly six-hundred-dollar paycheck in one night at different bars in Downtown Chicago.

There was a bar/restaurant in Chicago on the corner of Adams and Wells called King Arthur's Pub. This pub was famous for its yards of ale. A yard of ale or "yard glass" is a very tall beer glass used for drinking around two and a half imperial pints of beer, depending upon the diameter. The glass is approximately one yard long, shaped with a bulb at the bottom and a widening shaft, which constitutes most of its height. The yards at King Arthur's Pub also came with a very nice wooden holder. It was a classy place—at least it seemed classy for us. We would go to King Arthur's Pub on Fridays after work, which would be crowded with the downtown office crowd.

One particular Friday night, Jimmy and I sat down and ordered a "full yard" of beer apiece. The one yard of beer became three yards of beer each within an hour. Jimmy and I were enamored by the yards of beer. It got us drunker than regular glasses or bottles of beer. The beer went down your throat faster, and the whole presentation of the glass and the wooden holder were so utterly cool to us. We desperately wanted a yard for ourselves that we could steal and take home. Jimmy devised a plan and said to me, "Eddie, you run out the door with the yard. I will create some kind of distraction. Just keep running. Don't worry about me. You will figure out when to run." That made perfect sense to me. Don't ever mess with any of Piske's ideas, which always sound brilliant at the time.

Piske excused himself to go to the bathroom. I was just sitting on a couch in a daze, reeling from the three yards I had already consumed. The next thing I knew, I saw Piske running around the bar clutching and waving a live lobster in front of him and screaming like a lunatic. Piske had grabbed a live lobster from their aquarium and started to dance around with it, waving it around like a maniac. There were waiters and managers and bartenders trying to tackle him. Well, this must be my cue! I took off as fast as I could, yard in hand, right out the door and onto Wells Street. I immediately jumped on the train with my yard of beer and went home. When I woke up the next morning at my parents' house, I went downstairs and noticed the yard in our living room. My mom had filled it with M&M's—she had no clue that the real use of the yard was for beer, and I never had the heart to tell her. She did not approve of my drinking, and maybe my poor mom was trying to protect me the whole time.

The staff at the restaurant eventually let Piske go after they realized how drunk he appeared to be. Thank you very much, Jimmy. The plan went off without a hitch. I appreciate you.

That yard still sits in my condo. That yard puts a little smile on my face every time I see it. It reminds me of a time when drinking was fun and I did not have a worry in the world.

Wow, can life change.

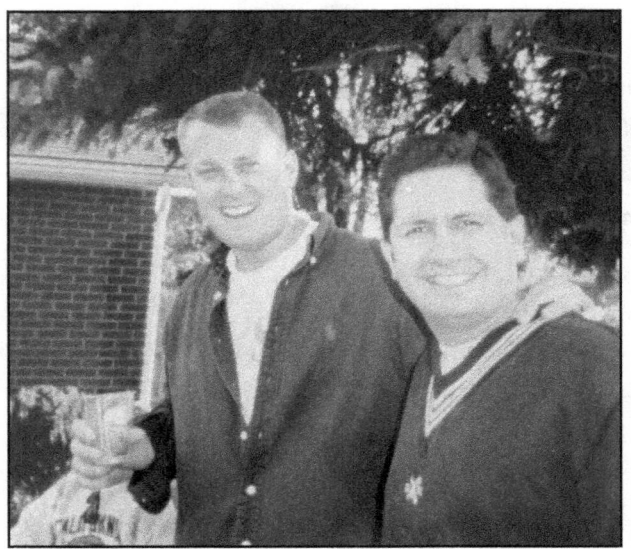

Me and the man, the myth, the legend—Jimmy Piske,
a great friend and drinking partner.

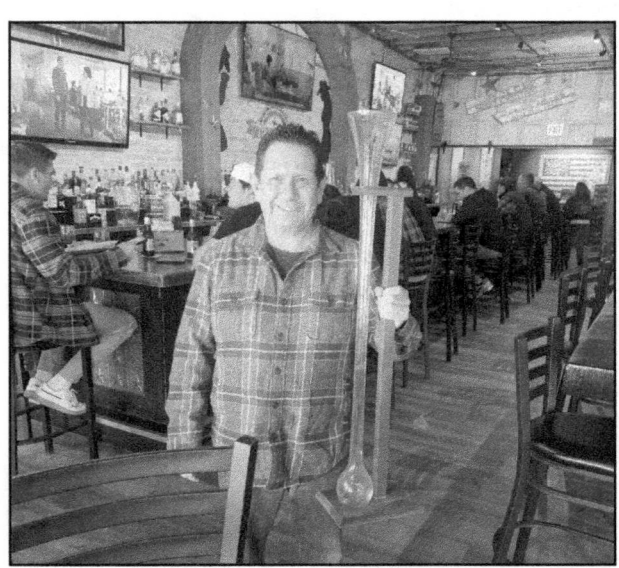

This was the actual yard that was stolen
from King Arthur's Pub in 1989

GETTING PUNCHED BY A SMALL FILIPINO WOMAN

February 1989

MY RECORD IN street fights is 0-16, which means that I have been involved in sixteen street fights in my lifetime and have lost all sixteen. I would say it is a safe bet to assume that I have not even been close to winning any one of them. I am not afraid to fight, however; I just am not very good at it, which is somewhat unusual considering how much mixed martial arts (MMA) and UFC-type fighting I watch on TV. It is also safe to assume that I have been very drunk during each one of these street fights. My voice gets very loud when I get drunk and I like to express my opinion quite loudly when I am hammered, which does not make for a perfect social situation.

I had been to the Chicago Blackhawks game at the Chicago Stadium downtown with Bill Pauly and Harry Carrold who were friends from work at the CME Audit Department. We went out right after work around 5 p.m. to various downtown bars. By the time we got to the Chicago Stadium, I was pretty fucked up. Considering the fact that I am a gigantic sports fan, it is pretty amazing how many games I have attended when I have been so drunk that I did not remember a single play or game.

After the game, we walked to a bar near the Chicago Stadium about three blocks away. It was very cold that night. I decided to urinate outside because the bathroom at the bar was too crowded. When I returned to the bar, Harry and Bill were nowhere to be found. They had fucking deserted me. I am sure I was too drunk to even remember them saying goodbye to me.

I didn't have much money on me (as I had spent it all at the bar), so I decided to take the Madison Avenue bus back to the Ogilvie train station so I could take a train home. I sat at the back of the crowded bus. A four-foot-tall Filipino woman boarded and sat right next to me. She did not speak English very well. We started a conversation—just shooting the shit. I loved speaking to strangers whenever I was drunk; I just didn't give a shit what I said or to whom I said it to. At one point during the conversation, I got up and started yelling at the small Filipino woman, "You stole my fucking watch! Give me my fucking watch back! You fucking stole my watch!"

My Movado watch, which had been given to me by my mom, was missing. This woman had for sure stolen it from me! I got right in this woman's face and demanded she return my watch. I had no idea how she could have gotten it off of my wrist, but you just don't think of shit like that when you are fucked up. The woman seemed very confused. She got up from her seat and proceeded to punch me right in the face with a left hook. Her father must have been a professional boxer, because she connected strongly. I immediately fell back in my seat as she ran toward the exit. Right before she exited the bus, she yelled, "Check in your pocket for your fucking watch!"

I was still reeling from the punch and in severe pain. I reached into my pocket, and sure enough, there was my watch. I must have taken my watch off so no one could steal it and put it in my pocket, and I must have told the Filipino woman about it. When I woke up the next morning, I had a huge black eye on the left side of my face. I had gotten the shit beaten out of me by a four-foot-tall, angry, Filipino woman. I should have stopped drinking from that moment forward.

This is the type of crazy shit that happened to me all the time. This was a clear sign that I couldn't handle alcohol. But, as in most of these situations, I thought it was a funny story, and I gladly told my friends the next day at work who thought it was hilarious. It is not so hilarious now. But at the time, I did not care. All I cared about was how much attention I could get from telling people my drinking story.

VALERIE VUARNET

September 1989

"**A MAN WILL** always be judged on the amount of alcohol he can consume. And a woman will be impressed, whether she likes it or not."

That quote was from the 1988 movie *Cocktail* starring Tom Cruise and Bryan Brown. Doug Coughlin, the veteran New York Upper-East-Side bartender was mentoring Brian Flanagan, the young up-and-coming bartender, with life quotes. I firmly believed every word of that quote. I was under the impression that women loved men who drank—and that they loved them even more if the men drank a lot.

One weekend, a few good friends and I went to a college football game at the University of Illinois at Urbana-Champaign. And I knew what that meant. There was zero interest in the football game for me. All I cared about was the fact that this was another perfect opportunity to drink as much as I wanted for as long as I wanted without anyone giving me any heat for it.

My recollection of the entire weekend is fuzzy at best. But certain aspects of it I do recall quite vividly. The second day we were there, I met a girl, Valerie Shay, at an outdoor barbecue. She was like someone out of a pin-up calendar—absolutely gorgeous. By some miracle of god, she was talking to me. Who knows what I was rambling on about because I was in one of those moods where I just talked and talked and probably repeated everything I was saying. Well, maybe she didn't realize how fucked up I was because she gave me her phone number.

I remember talking to her for about two and a half hours. The real time was probably about two and a half minutes. She was the only positive thing to come out of that weekend. When I got back to the CME office, I found out that a friend of mine, Dave Dejanovich, actually knew this woman. She had been Miss February of the University of Illinois's calendar the previous year. I had hit the jackpot! We had been communicating via phone (no texting back then). I would call her dorm room via a community phone, and someone would have to get her so we could speak.

During one of our conversations, Valerie complained that she had lost her sunglasses. Instinctively, I purchased a pair of Vuarnet sunglasses and I sent them to her via next-day delivery. Those Vuarnet sunglasses were expensive. Valerie Shay's name now changed to Valerie Vuarnet. Kind of has a nice ring to it, doesn't it?

Every year, the Chicago Mercantile Exchange used to have a fantastic holiday party at their building in Downtown Chicago. The party featured fantastic food, drinks, and entertainment. It was an extremely classy party. I invited Valerie Vuarnet to the party, which was on a Saturday night, and she said yes. Valerie was actually supposed to come into town on Friday. As luck would have it, my friends had organized a huge "Find Eddie a Wife" theme party at the Saratoga Bar and Grill located at Taylor and Loomis Street that night.

It might have been the party of the year. It ended with fights, the police, ambulances, hospitals, and stitches. I was told by my friends that Valerie Vuarnet had been at the party, but I do not remember seeing her, much less talking to her. She called me the following day, which was the day of the CME party. We talked for a little bit and she mentioned how drunk I had gotten and asked if I was okay.

I thought to myself: *Are you fucking kidding me? I get like that about three or four times a week! Wait till you see me tonight.*

I was supposed to pick her up at her parents' house in Northbrook, Illinois at about 7 p.m. for the CME party. I was all fired up for the evening, so I asked Jimmy Piske to go out with me for a few drinks that morning and afternoon to let off some steam. Piske and I had about ten drinks apiece. I got home at about 5 p.m. and decided to take a quick power nap before the party.

I woke up around 11:30 p.m. I saw about eight missed calls in my phone from a home in Northbrook. I called Valerie Vuarnet and explained to her that I had overslept and asked if she still wanted to go to the party. She declined and mentioned something about seeking help for my drinking. Well, I never heard from this "love of my life" ever again. I didn't understand why at the time. The nerve of her! The only times she had seen me, I was falling over and stupid drunk. I thought that was funny and impressive to women—wasn't it? What else could I have done with her? Taken her to dinner and then a movie? How the fuck was that "fun" for anyone?

It is funny how you look back in hindsight and realize how crazy your thinking was when you were drinking. A dinner and a movie would have been the perfect date. Maybe a woman didn't want to get black-out drunk as much as I did.

The truth is a woman is not impressed by how much a man can drink. Actually, women hate when men are drunk. I learned that the hard way. Unfortunately, I would continue to add to the long list of things I cared about that drinking "fucked up" for me a lot worse than when I was "fucked up."

HUMOR

Approximate Date: Ongoing

"EDDIE, THANK YOU for sharing."

"Eddie, that is powerful stuff."

"Eddie, that takes a lot of courage to write that about yourself."

"Eddie, you should write a book—those stories are amazing."

"Eddie, I love the stories, but I don't like all the f-bombs."

These people are referring to the drinking stories I had posted on Facebook during the fifteen-days lead-up to my sobriety date, and they were the impetus leading to writing this book.

I really appreciated anyone who took the time to read these stories and comment on them. They all really happened (at least from what I can remember of them and based on drunken eyewitness reports). Drinking is a subject that almost everyone is familiar with. Almost everyone reading this is affected by someone else's drinking—and 99.9 percent of the time, they are affected in a negative manner. Nobody has gone to AA because things were going great or because they were having too much fun or making too much money.

My all-time favorite movie is *Arthur*, starring Dudley Moore. The movie came out in 1981 when I was eighteen years old. I have seen the movie well over a hundred times. Dudley Moore plays the role of

Arthur Bach who is a drunk millionaire playboy living in New York City. I loved to have my friends come over to my house just to watch this movie. I can basically recite every line of the movie by heart. Arthur finds humor in almost everything he does, especially when he is drunk. I wanted to be him. I wanted to have all the money in the world and be perpetually drunk. Arthur Bach was one of my early role models in life.

I try to use humor in most or all of my drinking stories because it is a defense mechanism that I use to justify what I did or to make light of it so it doesn't sound so bad. A lot of hilarious things happen to people when they are drunk. The situations drunk people put themselves in are sometimes really funny. But there is always someone out there who is very close to you who does not think it is so funny.

Isn't it funny when a daughter is seeing her father yelling and swearing at her mother in a drunken rage and is scared to go to sleep?

Isn't it funny to sneak out of the house when your children are pleading for you to stay home and play Monopoly with them—while knowing that you were going out to get drunk?

Isn't it hilarious when you can only see your children every other weekend and one night a week?

Isn't it funny when your parents see you lying in a hospital room and your mother is crying uncontrollably because she thought you were dead?

Isn't it funny when you cannot answer the phone because you do not want to talk to anyone for fear of what happened the night before about which you cannot remember anything at all—but you know it was bad?

Isn't it funny to get fired from a job because you got there drunk at 7 a.m. and had to be escorted out by security?

Isn't it funny to be extracted from your car with the jaws of life after wrecking your car a block away from your house because you were passed out drunk at the wheel?

Isn't it funny when you discover that your community is laughing at you and not with you?

Isn't it funny to have a wife finding her husband sleeping on someone else's front lawn two blocks from their home at 9 a.m.?

Isn't it funny to be a child of an alcoholic?

Obviously, the answers to all of these rhetorical questions are a resounding no. The answers to these questions were not obvious to me at the time, though. I really believed that my drinking stories were funny. However, it really takes a lifetime of experiences, disappointments, and tragedies to truly understand why they are not funny. Most people have to find out for themselves.

I understand that alcoholism is not funny. I also understand that alcoholism can lead to the ultimate non-funny thing, which is death. My use of humor in retelling my drinking stories today is my way of escaping reality that alcohol use to do for me. I would rather be funny than be drunk at this point in my life.

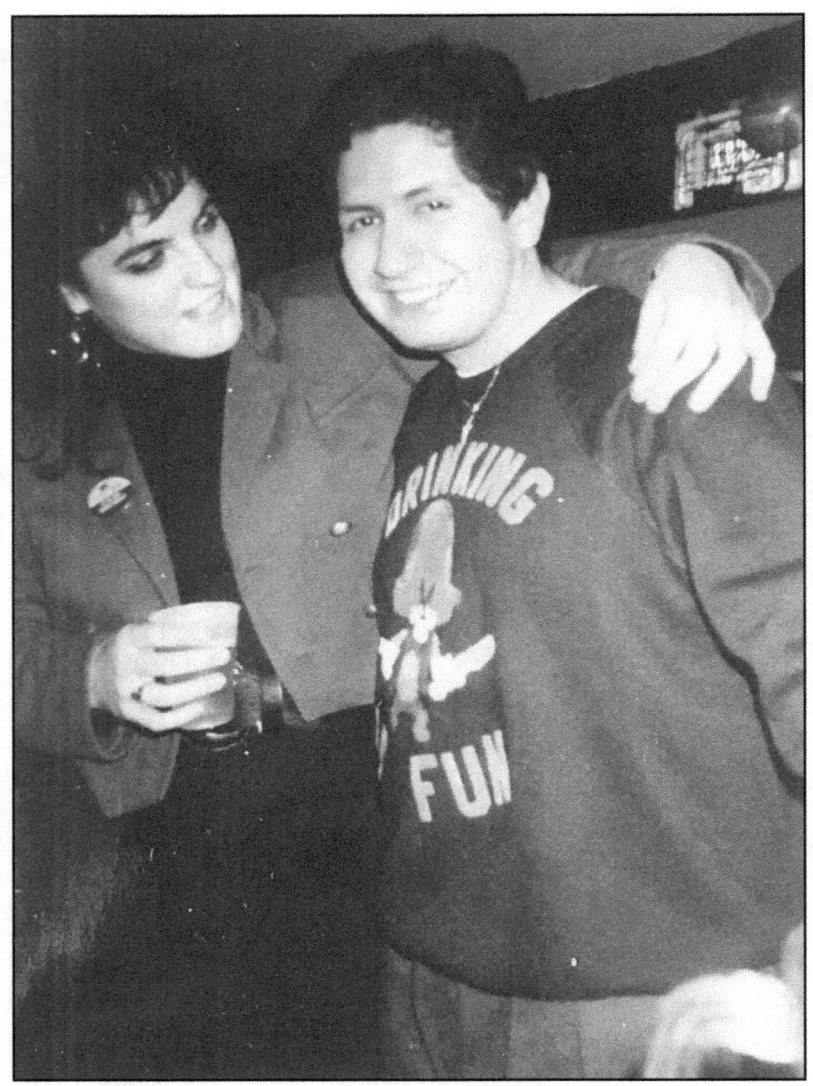

My friend Sheila Darcy and I, sharing a funny moment
while I am wearing my "Drinking Is Fun" sweatshirt.

THERESA CLAIRE WOLFE
(T. C.)

October 1988

"DID YOU GUYS see that girl from Marquette whom we interviewed today? I am going to marry her."

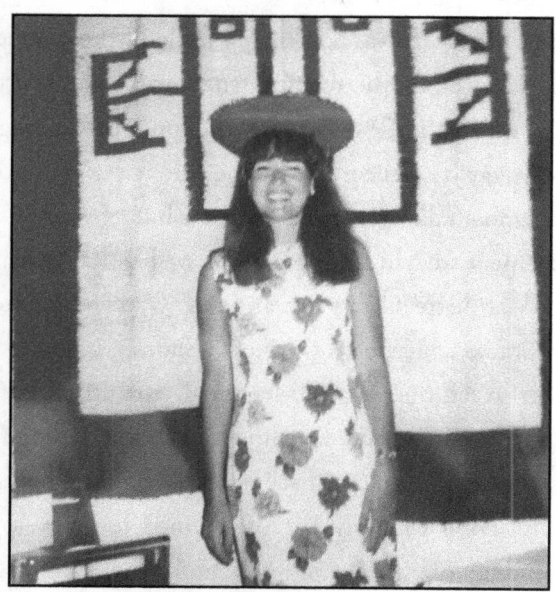

T.C. was forced to put on this Peruvian hat. She has always been a good sport!

I had been working at the Chicago Mercantile Exchange Audit Department for two years when our department decided to hire seven new auditors. Many of the people in our department were involved in the hiring and interview process. My particular job was to give the new job applicants a tour of the Chicago Mercantile Exchange trading floor. I was required to go on the actual trading floor and give them a tour of what was going on in the trading pits (of which I had no clue about) and provide a brief description of the staff auditor job. Shockingly, I was extremely hung over on that particular day. I barely made it to work that morning.

I had done my usual routine of copying blank pieces of paper in front of the bosses so they knew that I had shown up to work at an early hour. The first trading floor tour went very badly. I almost passed out on the floor of the exchange, and I did not like the candidate. He seemed like an arrogant asshole.

The second candidate was a woman. I took one look at her and was like "Woah, back the motherfucking truck up." I was smitten. I told her that I was way too hung over to take her onto the trading floor and asked if it was okay if I just conducted the "interview" from the visitor's gallery. I remember talking to her about how hung over I was and what a great department we had and how much we liked to party. She was a graduate of Marquette University and was from Wilmette, Illinois, a tony suburb near Chicago on the North Shore.

I asked her to tell the people from my department who had interviewed her that she had had a fantastic tour of the trading floor. I did not want my bosses to find out that I had been too hung over to do my job. She went along with my lie. She seemed to enjoy my sense of humor. I could not get her out of my head for the entire day.

Later on that evening, a bunch of guys from the office went to the Chicago Bulls game and we had a pre-party at a bar called Red Kerr's on Clinton Street. We were enjoying some beers and shots of whiskey before the game and talking about the new recruits whom we had interviewed that day. So, I announced to the group:

"Hey, do you guys remember that girl, T. C., from Marquette? I'm going to marry her."

Everyone just looked at me and laughed their asses off. They all remembered her and didn't think I had a shot in hell with her. T. C. Wolfe was eventually hired, and she started working at the CME Audit Department a few weeks later. As luck would have it, my desk was directly across from hers . . . c'mon, who am I bullshitting? I controlled the seating for this hire!

T. C. was what I referred to as a Triple Threat. She had looks. She had brains. She had a sense of humor. Most of the women I knew had only one of those qualities. A few girls had two of those qualities. But it was unheard of for a girl to have all three. She was a keeper. She was extremely social, and everyone liked her. She loved to go out after work and have drinks and socialize with other people from the department. This was perfect for me because I was the main organizer of the after-work crowd activities. T. C. and I became very close in a very short period of time.

Every day, I would get T. C. a present and put it on her desk before she arrived for work. I had endless stuffed animals, cards, supplies, bagels, donuts, coffees, jewelry, and clothes brought to her desk on a daily basis. I was a crazy motherfucker. When I want something—I want it. There was one minor problem, though. She was living with some guy in Highland Park, another rich-person suburb on the North Shore.

T. C. had a party at her apartment in Highland Park on a Saturday night and invited many people from work. I remember the party quite vividly. I was very impressed by how she lived and the style that she possessed. I wanted to be part of it. I was not used to shit like that. This was a life that I had no idea about. I knew she did not belong with the guy she was living with. He didn't treat her right. I noticed he was mean to her and constantly yelling at her. And I thought to myself, If this is how he treats her in public, I wonder how he treats her privately?

T. C. eventually moved out of Highland Park to Ravenswood (a North Side Chicago neighborhood) with this same guy about half a mile from my house, where I was living with my mom and dad. I would pick her up every day in my car, and we would drive to the train station and go to work together. T. C. showed me a whole new world that I had no idea existed. She taught me brand names of clothes. She taught me table settings. She taught me how to act in a country club. She taught me proper restaurant etiquette. She taught me the finer things in life. I was very impressed, and I wanted to be in that world that she had been her entire life.

T. C. and her boyfriend eventually broke up, and she moved to Presidential Towers in Downtown Chicago about a block away from the Chicago Mercantile Exchange. I was ecstatic. Eventually, I wore her down, and we started dating. Those early years of dating T. C. were the happiest years of my life. I knew that this was the woman I wanted to spend the rest of my life with. She tolerated me and thought I was funny.

On October 5, 1991, Edward Anthony Arana married Theresa Claire (T. C.) Wolfe at Faith Hope and Charity Church in Winnetka, Illinois.

I guess I wasn't so crazy when I told those guys at Red Kerr's that I was going to marry that girl from Marquette.

BETTY WOLFE: THE WILMETTE THREAT

November 1989

"WHO THE HELL are you?"

T. C. and I had gone to the Pumping Company on Broadway and Granville in Chicago on a Monday night. I was drinking Tanqueray (gin) and tonics and T. C. drank Miller Lite. We also played darts. It really did not matter what activity T. C. and I took part in. I really just enjoyed her company. At this point in my life, T. C. and I were still only work friends.

It was a work night, so we really couldn't overdo it on the drinking. Of course, I overdid it—immensely. We were not driving, and T. C. was going to spend the night at her mom's house in Wilmette, Illinois. I did not want her to take a cab by herself so I asked if I could join her. We got to her mom's house, and I started to dip into her scotch that was clearly on display to be consumed. Rumor had it that Betty, T. C.'s mom, also known as the Wilmette Threat, occasionally enjoyed a scotch or two when she had a chance to relax. I ended up passing out in the living room after way too many drinks.

In the morning, Betty walked downstairs and woke me up. She said, "Who the hell are you?" I explained to her that I was T. C.'s friend from work and that I hadn't wanted her to take a cab home by herself, so I joined her. Betty said, "I have heard a lot about you." She cooked me some wonderful scrambled eggs and bacon and gave me a tour of her fancy Wilmette house.

I was obsessed with a painting of a blue whale that T. C. had painted while she was in kindergarten. The bottom right was signed "Teacy." So I asked the Wilmette Threat, "What's up with that spelling of T. C.'s name?" She replied that "Teacy" was a secret spelling for Theresa Claire (T. C.) and that only close family members knew about it. And "Teacy" rhymes with "greasy"—so you'd know how to pronounce her name properly. Well, that was all I needed to hear. I now knew the secret spelling and the proper pronunciation of T. C.'s name.

Fast forward to September 1991:

T.C. and I eventually got engaged, and we had what is called a "couple's shower." I had no idea what this was, but I guessed it was a reason to drink and to get gifts for the wedding. We started opening up the many presents we had received and held them up so everyone could admire them. I had noticed a large present that was exquisitely wrapped in gold wrapping paper. I carefully opened it up, and to my amazement, it was the painting of the blue whale, framed, with the "Teacy" secret spelling!

Best present of the night! The Wilmette Threat had come through!

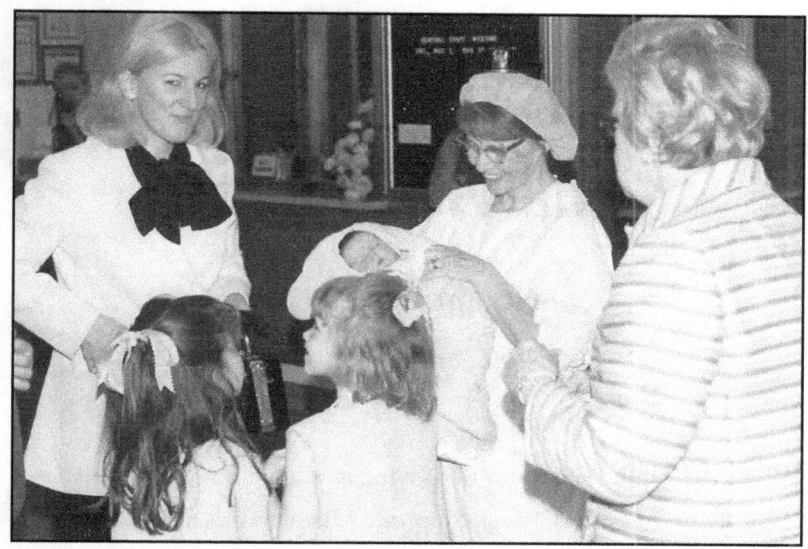

Betty Wolfe, the Wilmette Threat (far left), with T. C. (the dark-haired little girl) and her sister, Lisa (blonde-haired little girl).

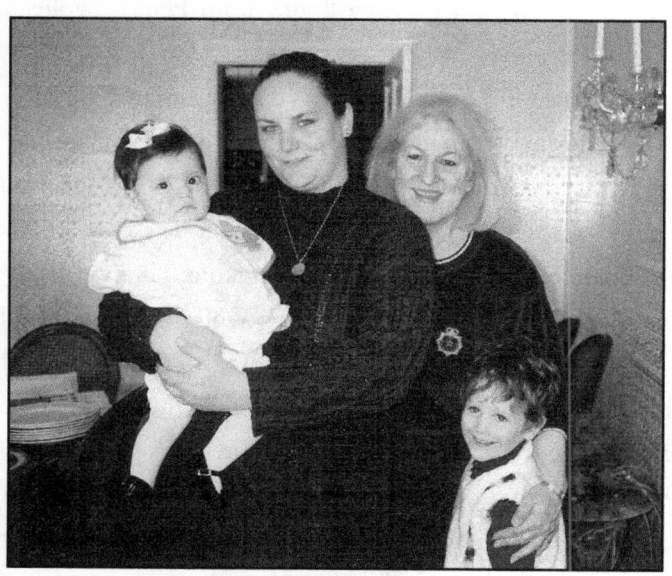

Betty Wolfe with her daughter Sarah, who is holding my daughter Sarah. Also pictured is Sarah's son, TJ.

FRANCIS WOLFE

November 1991

THE FIRST TIME I met him, I was lying facedown on his expensive rug in his living room in Chicago's upscale Lincoln Park neighborhood. I don't really remember how I got there. He started nudging at me and asked me to get up. I was startled and stood up. Then he extended his hand and said, "Hi, you must be Eddie. I am Francis Wolfe. It is a pleasure to meet you."

Francis Wolfe is T. C.'s father. To this day, he has been sober for over fifty years. He was a raging alcoholic and is famous for his line "Ten minutes to the bourbon!!" at the old Chicago Board of Trade. He made his fortune as a trader at the Chicago Mercantile Exchange and the Chicago Board of Trade. He would yell that famous line every day right before the grain markets closed. Francis Wolfe is known for being eccentric. He says and does off-the-wall things. Francis also traded at the old Chicago Butter and Egg Board in downtown Chicago. He claimed that there was a pole (similar to a fireman's pole) at this location that would take traders immediately from the trading floor to the bar below. Instead of racing to get to the fire, traders such as Francis would race to get to the bar.

He was quite a character, and I immediately liked him. Francis would eventually become my AA sponsor, but before that, we had some pretty wild times, including at my bachelor party, various meetings at gentlemen's clubs, and other crazy goings-on.

I asked Francis's permission to marry his daughter at the old Crazy Horse Gentlemen's Club on Kingsbury Street in Chicago. That was a glorious day. I gave him the address to where I wanted to meet him for a drink at 3 p.m. without telling him that the location was actually a gentlemen's club. I told him that there was something I needed to speak to him about. Francis was at a table when I arrived at 2:45 p.m. He was already talking to a dancer and having a great time. I got there and ordered a couple of drinks for myself and asked Francis if I could marry his daughter. Francis looked at me right in my eyes and smiled and said, "Yes, of course you can marry her!"

T. C.'s sister, Sarah, who was a high school kid at the time, had an impromptu party at his house in the early nineties. There must have been a hundred high school kids there from Wilmette, an affluent suburb in the city's North Shore. T. C. asked me to take a drive over there just to "check on things." That turned out to be a horrible mistake for T. C.—I ended up getting trashed at the party and then even moved the party to Glascott's Irish bar on Webster and Halsted. I vaguely remember Sarah bleeding and the cops showing up. The last thing I recall was passing out somewhere in Francis's house. Francis found me on his rug sometime the next morning. He never judged me or yelled at me. He just wanted to have a conversation with me and treated me like a human being.

Francis is a true drunk's drunk—a real pro. He went through the same things I eventually went through—divorce, facing the reality of no alcohol, and starting over. If you ever meet Francis Wolfe, you will never forget him. He is one of the funniest guys around and one of the most intelligent guys you could ever want to meet. He also has a very unique way of looking at life, as well as a sober way of looking at life. Yes, you can have that craziness in you and not drink. That is one of the things I most admire about Francis. One of the biggest compliments you can ever pay an alcoholic who is not drinking is "Wow, you are so great to be around when you are not drinking."

My number-one fear of not drinking used to be that I would no longer be social and would never be able to meet anyone. But I've found that just the opposite is true. I can meet so many more people when I am sober as opposed to when I am drunk. Women do not want to engage with someone who can barely stand up. I never really understood that concept back in the day, but now I understand it completely. It takes a lot of trial and error to fully comprehend, and I had a lot of trials that resulted in a lot of errors.

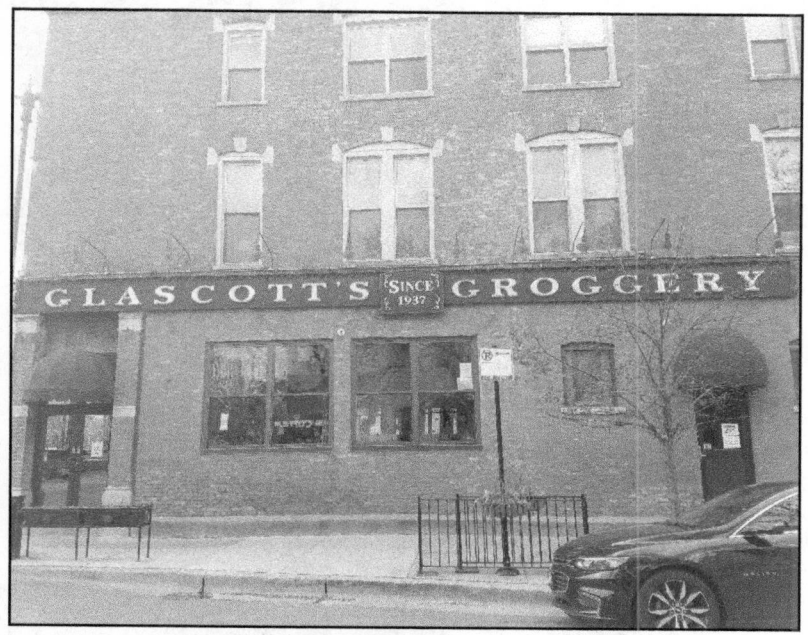

The bar across the street from Francis Wolfe's house
where I went drinking with T. C.'s sister, Sarah.

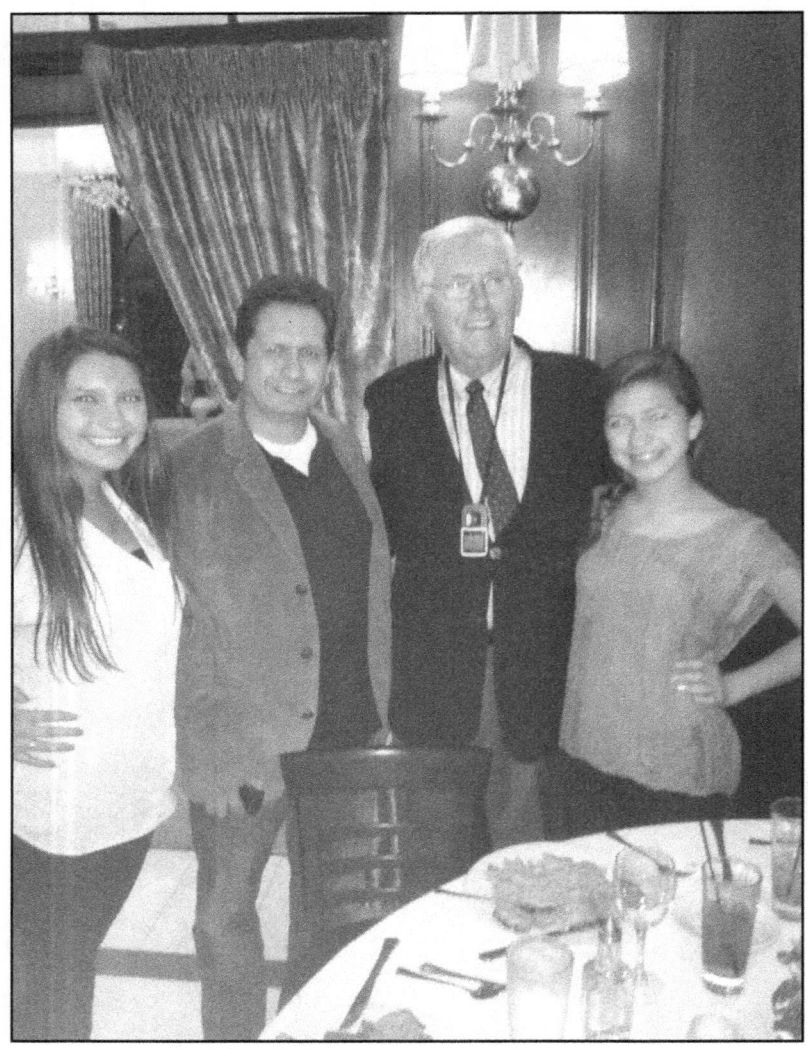

Pictured left to right: Sarah Arana, Edward Arana,
Francis Wolfe, and Isabelle Arana

GUILT

Approximate Date: Ongoing

GUILT IS A big part of my life now.

I feel guilty for falling asleep and snoring at my daughter Sarah's first piano recital when she was seven years old and getting thrown out of the church.

I feel guilty for not taking my son to a baseball game because I was too hung over; I told him I was "sick" and still went out later that day and got hammered again.

I feel guilty for urinating all over myself at a CME-sponsored Cubs game outing and telling my daughter that it had "rained" during the game when I stumbled home.

I feel guilty for putting my parents through hundreds of days and nights of wondering if I was ever going to come home; or which bus stop or park bench they had to guess I was sleeping on; or which hospital they had to pick me up from after I was treated for stitches; or whose house they had to pick me up and carry me out the door from; or if their son was going to make it through the night alive.

When you are young, you truly think you are invincible. Nothing that you do can hurt you. You can drink as much as you want—and you know that somehow you will get home and you will never get hurt and you will never die. Only once you become a parent do you realize and truly fear what can happen to your children when they are "out there," as they say in AA.

My parents were the nicest people in the entire world. They did not deserve the torture that I put those poor Peruvians through. I gave zero fucks when it came to them. I didn't give it a single thought growing up. All I wanted to do was get fucked up.

Once that little seed is planted in your head, it takes your life over. I suppose that it really isn't someone's fault if you believe in the "disease" part of alcoholism. But you certainly have a choice. You do not have to go out. You can stay home. You can be with your children or you can stay with your wife. However, once you put yourself in that situation when you feel the urge, there really is no choice. You just do it. It is a very weird sensation that you cannot control, or at least you feel you cannot control it.

I DRANK APPLE JUICE AT MY WEDDING

October 5, 1991

THERE WAS ONLY one day I recall in my "drinking history" that I made a conscious decision not to drink, and I stood by it. I drank apple juice on October 5, 1991—my wedding day. Deep down in my heart, I was probably already aware then that I was an alcoholic. I hated the taste of alcohol, especially beer, yet I would think nothing of drinking twelve to eighteen beers in a single sitting. But I loved the taste of apple juice.

I really enjoyed going through my parents' wedding albums from the year 1960. The expressions on people's faces were priceless. The whole world seemed like such a happy place. The black-and-white pictures in the church mesmerized me. Their wedding was magical. It was something that I wanted to replicate.

I did not want to embarrass my children or myself when people saw our wedding album. Maybe way back then, I recognized my alcoholism, even if for just one day, and I did something about it. I have never gone back and regretted that day and said, "Damn, I wish I would have gotten fucked up that day."

I chose to drink apple juice the entire day and night. I did not have one drop of alcohol on my wedding day. I equated alcohol with bad and apple juice with good. And I wanted the most important day of my life to be good. I knew that we would have children one day, and I did not want them to think their dad was bad and a drunk.

Letter to my children:

Your dad is an alcoholic. Your dad is a drunk. He just wasn't drunk on his wedding day.

I am truly sorry that I wasn't the man or father that I should have been throughout all those years when you were growing up. I wish I would have had the same thought process when you were growing up that I had on my wedding day.

Sarah, I am so sorry I fell asleep during your first piano recital and got kicked out of the church. I am sorry doe throwing your cupcake in the high school parking lot because you were afraid of the costume the GT mascot was wearing.

Eddie, I am so sorry for not going to enough baseball games with you. I am so sorry for not helping you with your homework. I am so sorry for going out drinking even after you begged me to stay home.

Isabelle, I am sorry that I fell asleep during your gymnastics meets. I am sorry for driving you around drunk on many occasions. I could have killed you. I am sorry.

T. C., I am sorry that I was a horrific husband and drank my way through our marriage. You deserved better.

I drank apple juice at my wedding. At least there isn't an embarrassing story about that day.

GOOD THINKING, EDDIE.

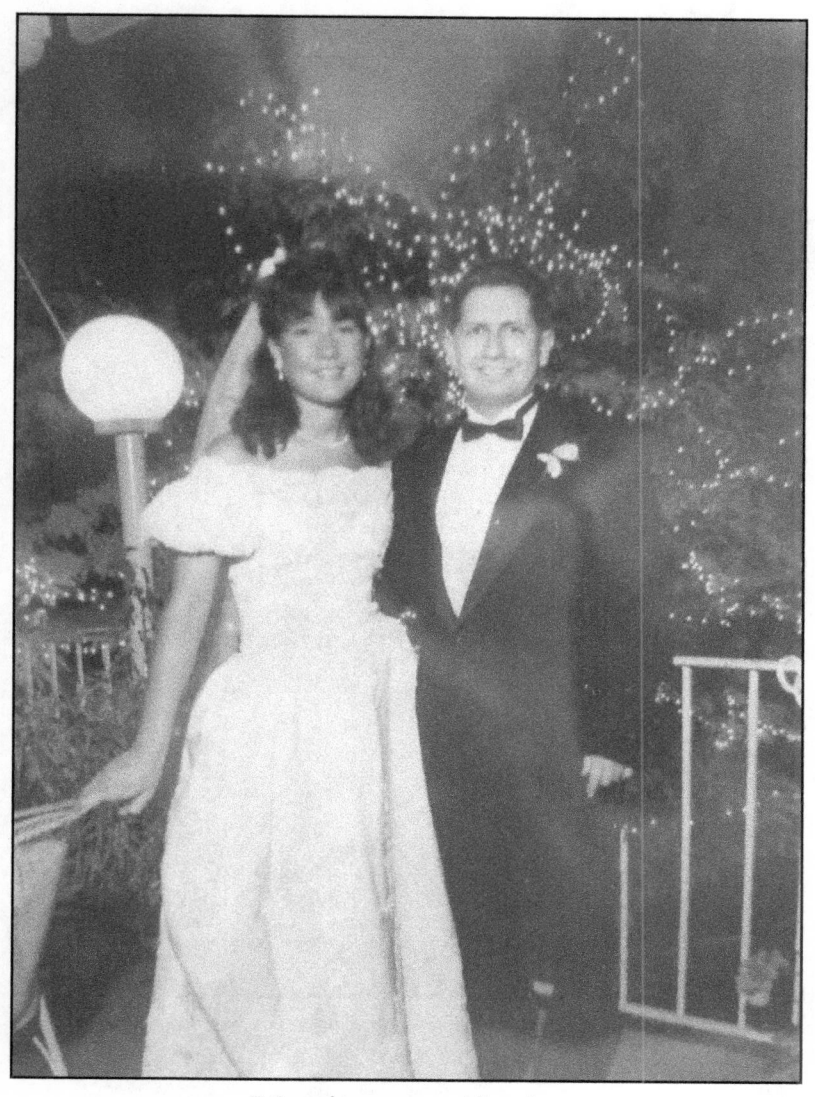

T. C. and I on our wedding day.

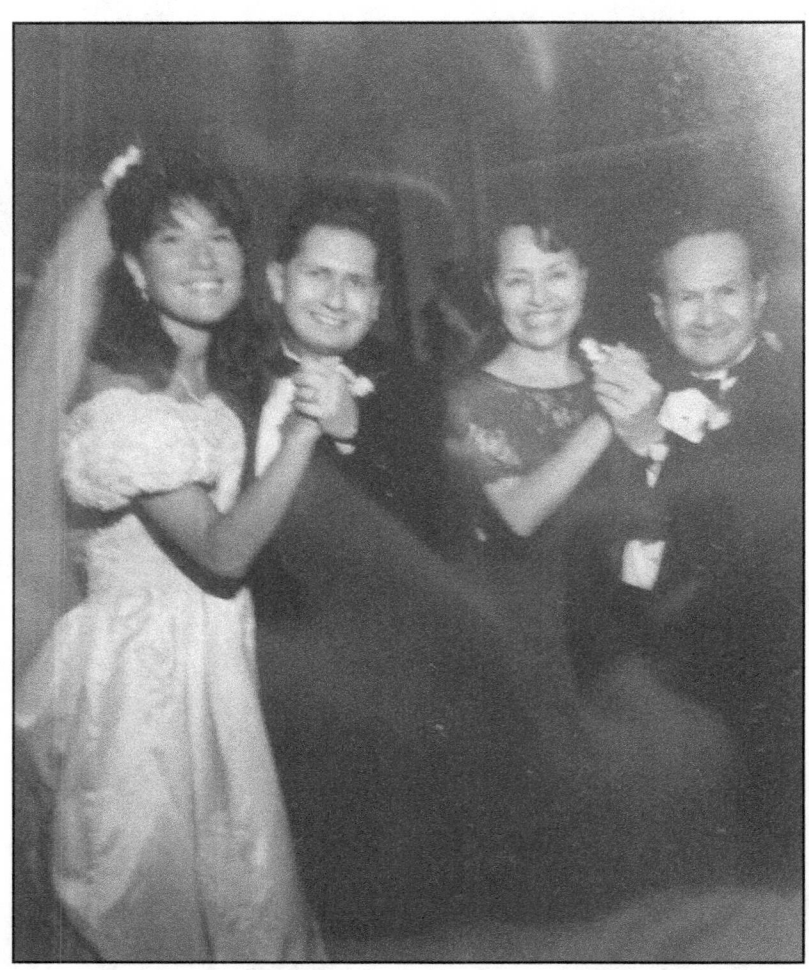

T. C. and I and my parents dancing at my wedding.

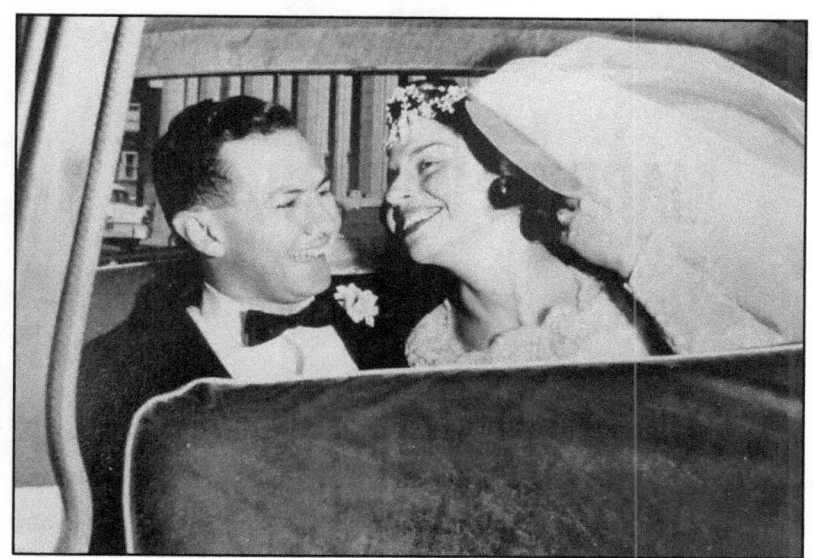

My parents in their limo after their wedding.

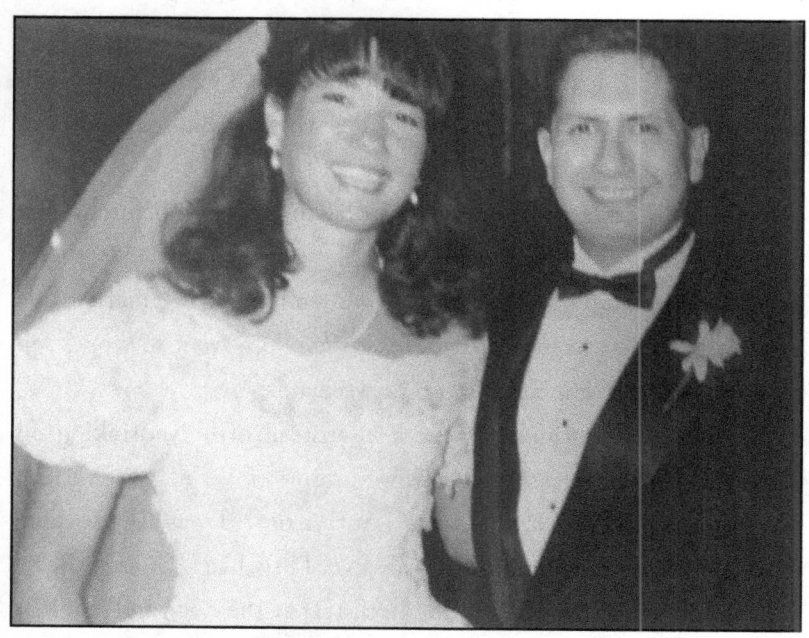

My wedding day—I remember it all—thanks to the apple juice.

MARRIED WITH NO KIDS

October 1991 to September 1993

T. C. AND I lived in a two-bedroom apartment on the third floor on Northwest Highway in Chicago's Edison Park neighborhood. This was a neighborhood that consisted mostly of police, firefighters, and city workers who were required to live in the city of Chicago. We would take the train together into downtown every day to go to work. I could have lived in that apartment for the rest of my life. I was so happy with cable television, steak dinners, and living within walking distance of the bars.

T. C. and I never really talked about having children before we got married. I just went with the flow. If T. C. wanted to have kids, then I guess we were going to have kids. I was really enjoying married life without kids. Life seemed so easy back then. You went to work, you made money, and you had fun on the weekends.

My drinking continued to escalate. Instead of only drinking on weekends, I would occasionally throw a couple of weekday nights into the mix disguised as "work outings." At this time, I was also working once a week at the Pumping Company. They had "Quarter Beer" nights every Wednesday. I would check IDs at the door and drink as much beer and shots as I wanted.

Here are a few examples of the shenanigans I was involved in during this time in my life:

I was on a business trip to New York City with my colleagues Jack Bouroudjian and John Ringer. We had gone to a gentlemen's club, Scores, the previous night and were flying back to Chicago first thing in the morning. Our flight was at 7:30 a.m. and we had gotten back to our hotel rooms around 5 a.m. We barely made it on time to LaGuardia airport to catch our flight. In the airplane, I needed to take a shit very badly. In my still-drunken state, I forgot to take off my underwear during the defecation process. During the two-and-a-half-hour flight, I sat in my seat with my underwear packed with about two pounds of fresh shit. My entire row moved out of their seats because they could not stand the stench.

I had gone to lunch with my boss at the Billy Goat Tavern in Downtown Chicago. Part of my work responsibilities included sending bank wire transfers every day by 3:30 p.m. After drinking about ten pitchers of beer over a three-hour period, I stumbled back to the office and sent the wire transfers just in the nick of time. When I came in to work the next morning, I discovered that instead of sending out a wire transfer for two hundred thousand dollars ($200,000), I had mistakenly sent out the wire transfer for two hundred million dollars ($200,000,000). Our company bank account was overdrawn for the night. It was a gigantic mistake on my part. I'm not exactly sure why I was not fired for this egregious error.

LESSON: DO NOT DRINK AND BANK.

I was at Olympic Gardens, a strip club in Las Vegas, attending my friend Yaki's bachelor party. We had a separate private party area roped off for our entire group. I had been drinking scotch for two days straight and was extremely drunk. On one of my many trips to the bathroom, I became disoriented and ended up in the middle of another private party. This party was hosted by actor Sylvester Stallone. I made an attempt to introduce myself and talk to him, and I was quickly whisked away by his security staff. I started yelling quotes from his movies at the top of my lungs, such as:

"Hey Tango, where's Cash?" (*Tango and Cash*)
"Yo, Adrian!" (*Rocky*)
"Hey, Cobretti, I just want to drink with you!" (*Cobra*)
"He drew first blood!" (*Rambo*)

I was escorted out of the club by security amidst the cheers of all my friends who had gathered around the spectacle I had created.

T. C. and I were vacationing in New Orleans with my friend Steve Brewer and his girlfriend, Cheryl Ann Arts, for a long weekend. Steve and I had already been drinking since we stepped foot in O'Hare airport in Chicago for our flight. On our first day, the girls spent the entire day at the pool while Steve and I were at the bar at the hotel. We then had a lavish dinner at Emeril's Delmonico restaurant on St. Charles Avenue. Steve drank Grey Goose vodka and I enjoyed Glenlivet scotch. After dinner, we went to Pat O'Brien's in the French Quarter for their world-renowned hurricanes. T. C. and Cheryl Ann were so tired from the long day that they went back to the hotel. Steve and I went to a strip club, whose name I have never figured out to this day. I woke up in the bathroom of the strip club at 7:30 a.m. to a total of fifteen missed calls from T. C. As I started my one-mile walk back to the hotel, I spotted Steve Brewer, who had apparently fallen asleep in some kind of VIP room at the strip club and was walking home, too. T. C. was furious when I got back to the hotel room.

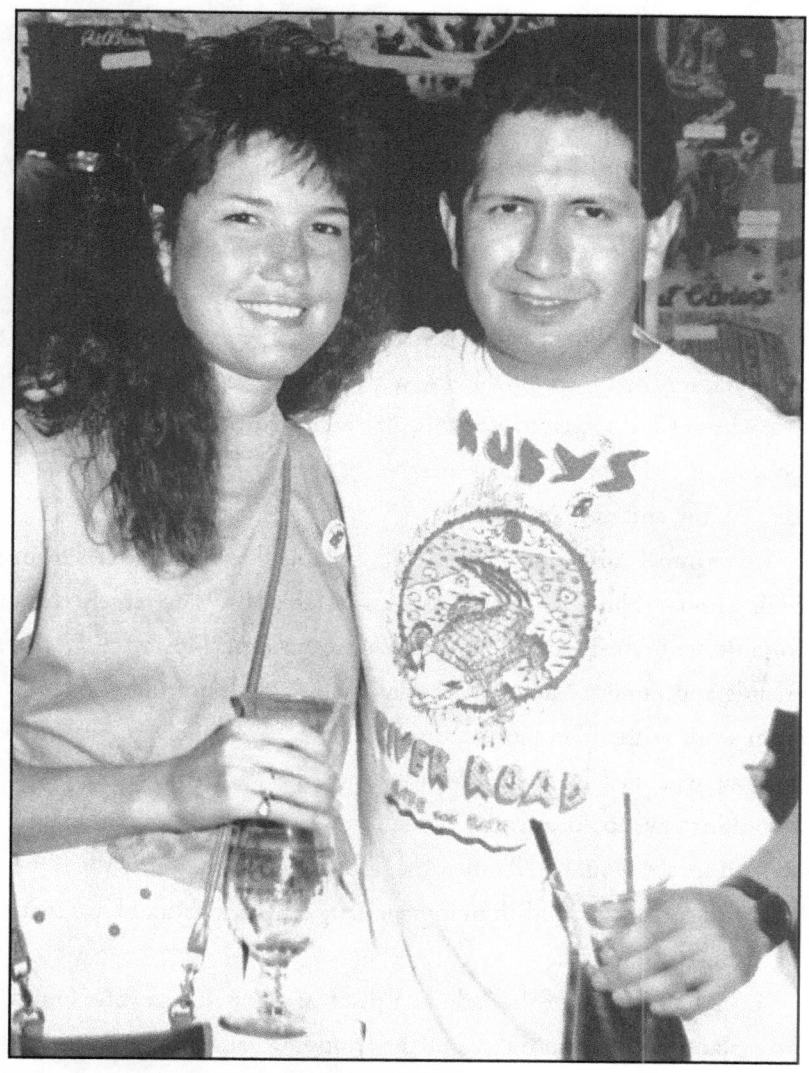

T. C. and I enjoying hurricanes at Pat O'Brien's in New Orleans.

The night before Thanksgiving was always the biggest bar night for kids who were in college and were home for the holidays. It was no different for me. I had gone to work at the Pumping Company and had gotten so drunk that a friend from the bar had to drive me home. I invited my friend Angel up to my apartment to continue drinking at about 4 a.m. T. C. and I had invited my parents and her mom (the Wilmette Threat) over for Thanksgiving dinner later that day. This was also the first time T. C. had attempted to make a turkey, which was already made and sitting in the kitchen. Angel and I were so drunk and hungry that we started to eat the turkey and all of the fixings. T. C. woke up and threw Angel out of the apartment.

Again, my drinking patterns remained the same. A major difference, however, was that I was now living with a wife. I was living with some- one whom I had vowed to stay with "for better, for worse; for richer, for poorer; in sickness and in health . . . " I cannot truthfully say that I kept up my end of the bargain.

I continued to go out with my old, reliable drinking buddies from high school—Nino, Milazzo, Piske, and Marco. I was extremely com- fortable with them. I had also developed relationships with T. C.'s friends and family. I had strong relationships with newfound friends from work at the Chicago Mercantile Exchange Audit Department. I was overwhelmed by the number of people I wanted to drink with. I couldn't say no to anyone. Sometimes T. C. would join me, and sometimes she wouldn't. At the time, it didn't really matter to me if she was with me or not, and thinking back on things, it should have mat- tered the world to me.

T. C. handled all of the "adult" aspects of our marriage. She found us a place to live. She did all of the shopping. She was an awesome interior decorator. She paid all of the bills. She made me go to family events. She made me do things with my own family that I did not want to do. T. C. was an adult, and I really was not.

I was still yearning for that first feeling I'd had when I drank my dad's Chivas Regal in their basement on Hermitage. I craved a buzz like that one. You chase that buzz for years and years before you realize that it will never happen again. Hopefully, you can figure that out before disaster strikes for you.

I was also still chasing clout. Drinking made me extremely popular to everyone—or at least I thought it did. I still wanted to create that scenario where my drinking escapades would be talked about for years to come. I wanted my drinking to be known as "legendary." I sought and craved that drinking affirmation more than anything. I definitely craved it more than I craved having a happy marriage.

Marriage is a lot of work.

Whoever came up with that saying is a genius. If you do not work at your marriage, it will fail. I was a prime example of that. I didn't have a clue of what it meant to be a good husband. And I would soon learn that I didn't have a clue of what it meant to be a good father.

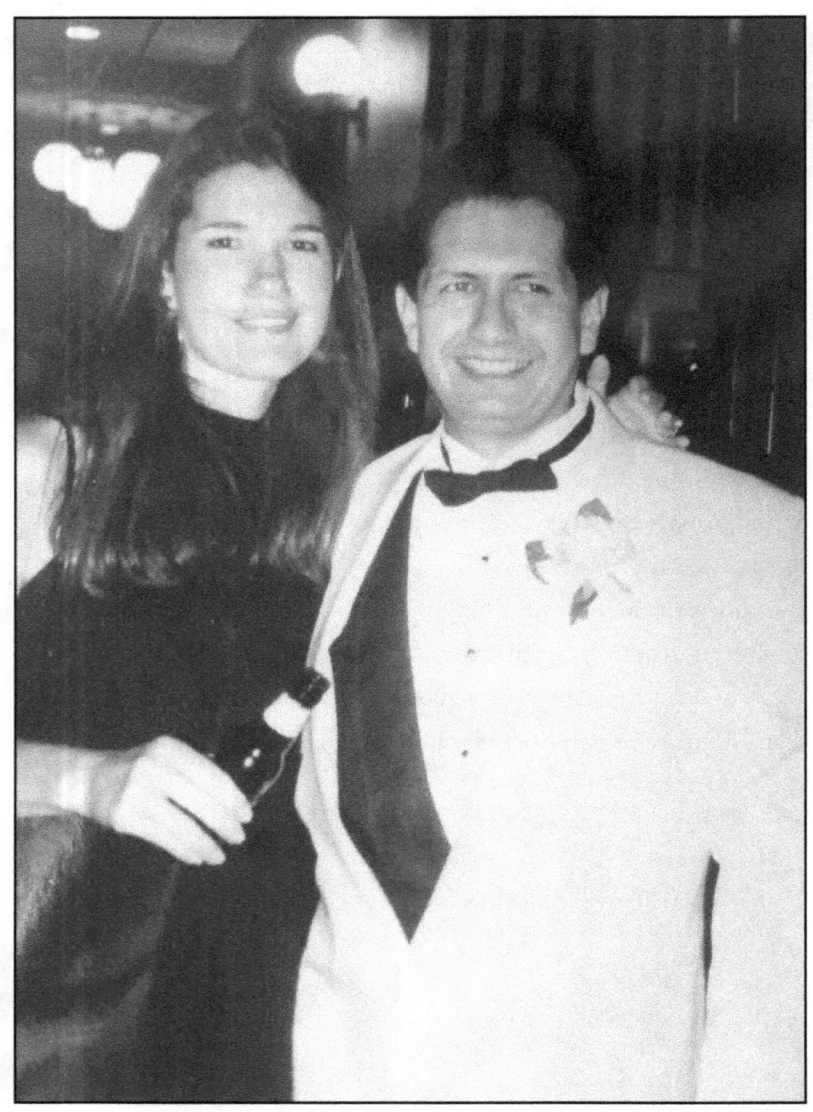

T.C. and I at Yaki's wedding

MY MISTRESS KILLED MY MARRIAGE

October 5, 1991

I CHEATED ON my wife for about thirteen out of the fourteen years we were married. I was twenty-nine years old when I got married. I had met my mistress/girlfriend when I was about sixteen years old or so. We hit it off right away, and I never really got over her. She was the best. I fell in love with her the instant I met her. I just wanted to see her every day and every night. I had never met anyone who was so vibrant and who knew what to say and when to say it. She was fantastic in social situations, and she had all kinds of energy. She was also a fantastic dancer.

We dated all through college and into my early work years. My wife (at the time) had actually met her on several occasions, but I don't believe she knew the full extent of our relationship. I am sure she never would have married me if she had. What woman in her right mind would marry someone who is in love with someone else? When I was married, I tried to leave my girlfriend on many, many occasions. Every one of my efforts to leave was unsuccessful.

This mistress just kept coming back to me, and it seemed like she just got better looking every day. I mean, she was like a supermodel to me on certain days. She was very easy to get along with, as well. We never had to talk about taking care of the kids. We never had to talk about money issues. We never had to talk about things that really mattered. All she wanted to do was have a good time. And I just loved the idea of having a good time.

Well, to make a long story short, my wife finally found out the true nature of my relationship with my mistress. I couldn't hide her any longer. It was extremely hard to maintain a marriage, have three kids, and have a full-time mistress who needed my attention all the time. Sadly, my wife and I got divorced. My mistress didn't seem to really care, though. She just kind of went about her own business.

She hurt me really bad. I wanted to be with her forever, or so I thought.

I finally ended the affair with my mistress. It just wasn't worth it to me anymore. She still texts me every single day without fail. It is so difficult to say no to her. But sometimes, you just have to grow up and do the right thing. I am sure she is just fine.

I heard she is dating a good friend of mine.

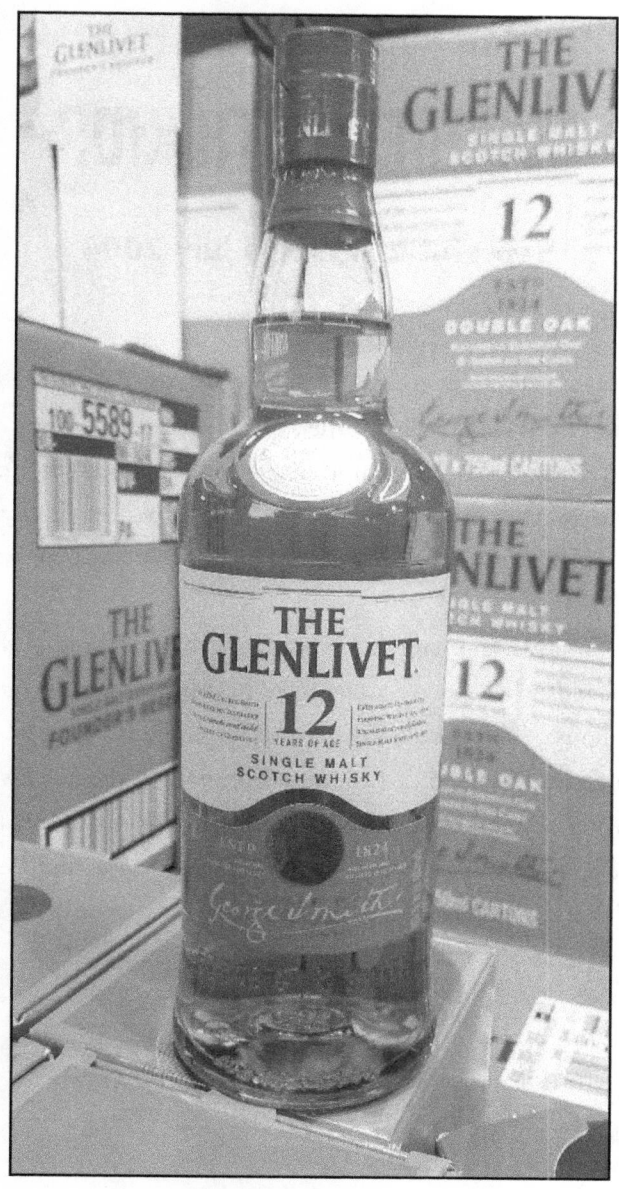

My Mistress for 15 years of marriage

MARRIED WITH KIDS

September 1993 to July 2004

I THOUGHT I was ready to be a father. I had a decent job. I was married to a great woman. We lived in a great neighborhood—the "country club" area in Park Ridge, Illinois. We had a perfect family. Sarah was born in 1993, little Eddie was born in 1995, and Isabelle was born in 1999.

I had fantastic and supportive parents. My mom and dad would watch the kids whenever we asked them to. My kids loved to go to my parents' house. They got whatever they wanted at 5251 W. Argyle Street in Chicago's Jefferson Park neighborhood on the northwest side of the city. T. C. and I felt so comfortable dropping them off there so we could go out and have fun. Our kids were happy and healthy. I thought that was all that was important in life.

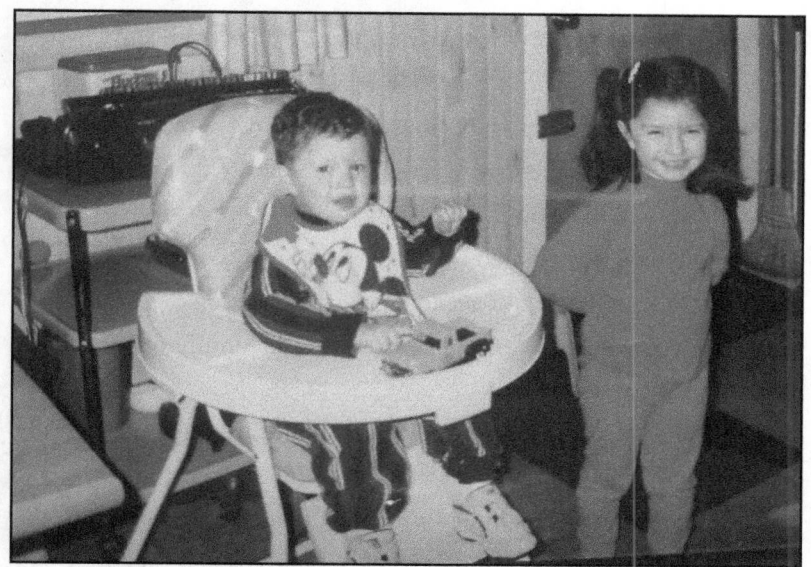

Sarah and little Eddie at my parents' house at 5251 W. Argyle.

However, I had this dirty little secret. I could not drink normally. I could not just have "a couple of drinks." I had to take it to the next level. Sometimes, I could control it and drink like a normal person. But sometimes, I could not control it and I was off to the races. The problem with alcoholism is that you cannot predict which person you are going to be that day. And the bigger problem is that your problem will only continue to get worse. You do not all of a sudden become a "normal" drinker. I wish it were that easy. And I wish I had addressed this issue way before I was forced to address it.

I was a master manipulator, especially toward my wife, T. C. I really thought I was getting away with it every time I explained to her why I needed to go out with my friends. Typically, I would plant the seed between 1 and 4 p.m., and I would make up some controversy or emergency that one of my crazy friends was involved with and say they needed my help.

"Nino needs my help. His brother is talking about burning his house down. He wants me to go over there. I really don't want to go. Hopefully, it will blow over."

After the seed was planted and watered a bit throughout the day, I would get in the shower and get changed and get ready to go out. T. C. would ask me where I was going, and I would simply respond with something like this:

"I'm going to Nino's house. I told you about this. I guess they really need my help."

At this point, my exit strategy was fully mapped out. Hopefully, the kids would have already been put to bed. I hated when they were still up because the guilt I felt about going out and leaving them with T. C. really bothered me. It never bothered me enough not to go out, but it definitely bothered me. I always felt like I had gotten away with something. I never wanted to look T. C. directly in the eyes during one of these "escapes" because I did not want to see the hurt I knew I had caused.

Every night was the same. I would come home so drunk that I didn't know who I was or where I had been. The following day, I would be of little to no help in doing anything with T. C. or the kids. I was too "tired" to engage with anyone. I really thought that was normal behavior for a husband and father. Deep down, I probably knew that I should have done much more, but when that alcoholism has a grip on you, it is very difficult to let it go.

Here are three more examples of how out of control I was with a wife and three kids at home wondering where I was and what time I would be home:

My friend Tommy Pinsky had season tickets for the Chicago Bears. He loved to tailgate near Soldier Field for every home game. He honored me by asking me to go to a game with him on a particular Sunday. He picked me up at 6 a.m., and I had drunk a bottle of Glenlivet by 7:30 a.m. I loved to drink early in the morning—especially at events where it was socially acceptable to drink that early. Tailgate parties were perfect occasions for me. I could drink as much as I wanted and no one could or would say a word to me. This was a drinker's paradise. When it seems like everyone around you is drinking to excess, for a drinker, it just appears like you are fitting into societal norms. At least for a few hours, you are drinking just like the rest of the crowd. It is just another way alcoholics justify their drinking.

I continued to drink until 11:30 a.m., and then we proceeded to walk about a mile and a half to the stadium. I had brought my all-time favorite Chicago Bears hat—a blue, furry, helmet-like hat that I treasured. Another fan admired my hat and offered me thirty dollars for it. I quickly accepted his offer. Keep in mind—I adored that hat. I was the biggest Bears fan in history and had had that hat for at least twenty years. What could have possibly convinced me to sell my hat to a complete stranger? Why did I do that? Soon afterward, I defecated all over myself and never made it inside the stadium. I smelled like a dirty barn. I took a cab home and missed the entire game and passed out at home. My kids and wife were scratching their heads wondering what had happened to me. Tommy Pinsky chastises me to this day about the hat incident, and it's yet another reminder of the illogical things alcohol made me do that seemed to make sense at the time.

On September 16, 2002, Steve Brewer and I had the chance to see the Rolling Stones at the Aragon Ballroom. We each paid a thousand dollars per ticket for this opportunity of a lifetime to see a legendary band in a relatively small venue (it had a capacity of about five thousand people). Our friend Max Waisvisz, who owned Gold Coast Tickets, walked us into the VIP balcony area. Steve and I had been drinking since 2 p.m. All kinds of celebrities were in the VIP area. Steve was talking to Bono from U2 at one point in the night. While I was waiting in line for the bathroom, I started drinking from a small bottle of Jack Daniel's that I had with me. I was immediately grabbed by Aragon Ballroom security and taken to the Aragon "jail" located in the basement of the building. This "jail" was meant for unruly guests who had too much to drink or who appear to be incoherent for some other reason. I spent the rest of the night in "jail" and missed the entire concert.

Nino Speciale and I met at the Bucktown Pub on Courtland and Paulina Street in Chicago's Bucktown neighborhood. I drove my Chrysler 300 that night for some stupid reason. I hardly ever drank and drove, but I did that night. I also had a bottle of blackberry brandy in my pocket, which was finished by the end of the night. At about 2 a.m., Nino asked me if I was okay to drive. I looked at him like he was crazy, and off I went into the night. On the Kennedy Expressway, I must have fallen asleep at the wheel, and I was involved in a three-car pileup. Multiple police were at the scene. By some miracle of god, a state policeman whom I had known from Gordon Tech High School was on the scene. He called an ambulance for me and had my car towed to my parents' house. I received three stitches above my left eye and was free to go home. I did not receive a DUI. I had dodged another bullet.

After I got sober, my friend Joel and I would talk about alcoholism on a daily basis. He would constantly harp on the old AA saying that alcoholism is not really about the actual drinking but rather about "the thought that precedes the first drink." I could not summarize alcoholism into a better concept than that.

My alcoholism was solidified every morning when I woke up and planned my day. If I knew that I was going out drinking that day or night (the thought that precedes the first drink), my entire morning or afternoon would be entirely dedicated to getting whatever I needed to get done in order to drink that afternoon or night. I would create a daily to-do list so I would not forget anything. I never wanted to get "caught." I did not want anyone to think that my drinking impacted my life in a negative manner.

I even started running in order to convince myself and others that I did not have a problem. If I ran a marathon, then I couldn't possibly have a drinking problem, right? I ran two marathons while I was married. I wanted to protect this drinking problem so badly. I even ran when I was so hung over that I could barely wake up. I had to protect this secret at all costs. Every morning at 5:30 a.m., I would go on my daily five-to-ten-mile run—no matter what.

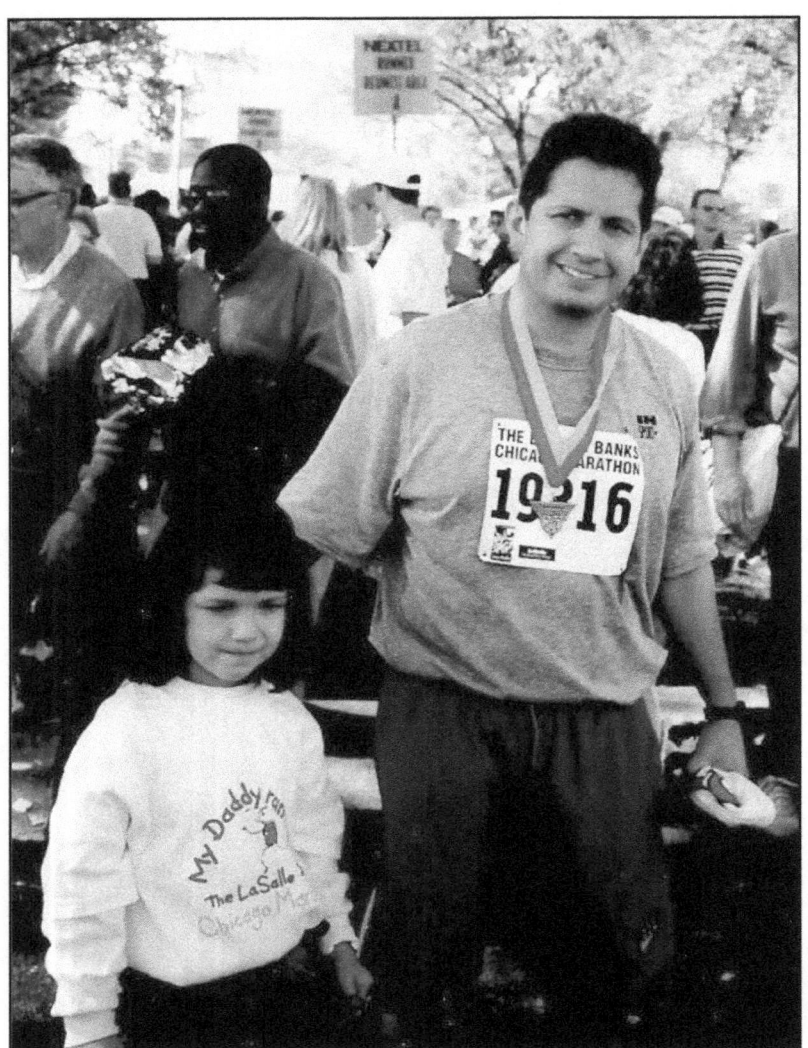

Sarah and I at the 1996 Chicago Marathon.

Let us assume that I did not plan to drink on a particular day. I would receive a phone call from my buddy, Jimmy Piske. All he had to say was some sort of remark about how much we loved a particular bar or how great it would be to see a particular person—and boom! The thought that precedes the first drink would now be in my head. And there is nothing that you can do to stop it. It is like a runaway train. Your mind has been so well trained that the only thing that can satisfy this never-ending mental thirst is to have a drink.

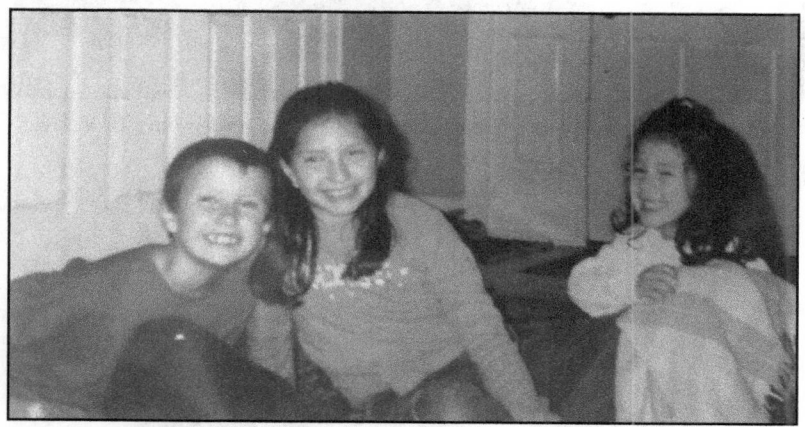

Little Eddie, Sarah, and Isabelle at our home in Park Ridge.

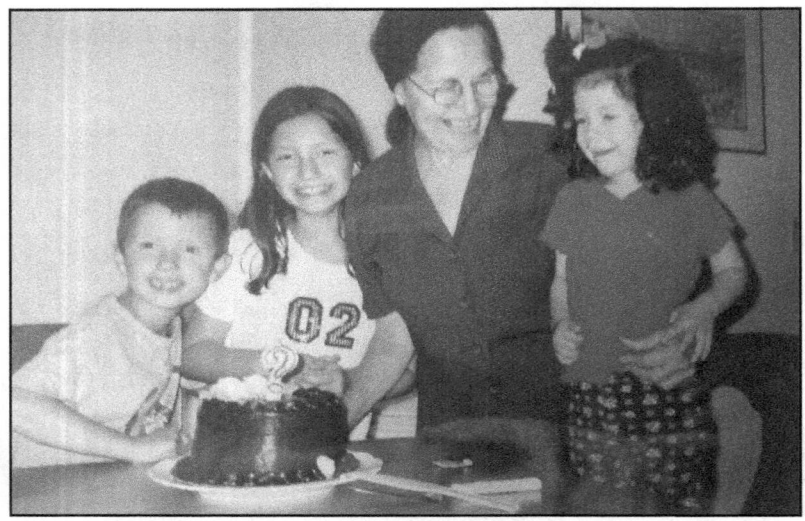

Little Eddie, Sarah, my Mom, and Isabelle celebrating my mom's birthday.

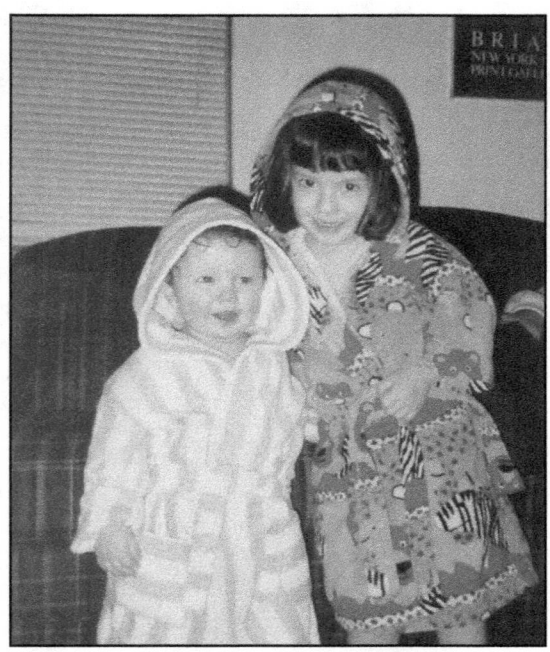

Little Eddie and Sarah ready for bath time.

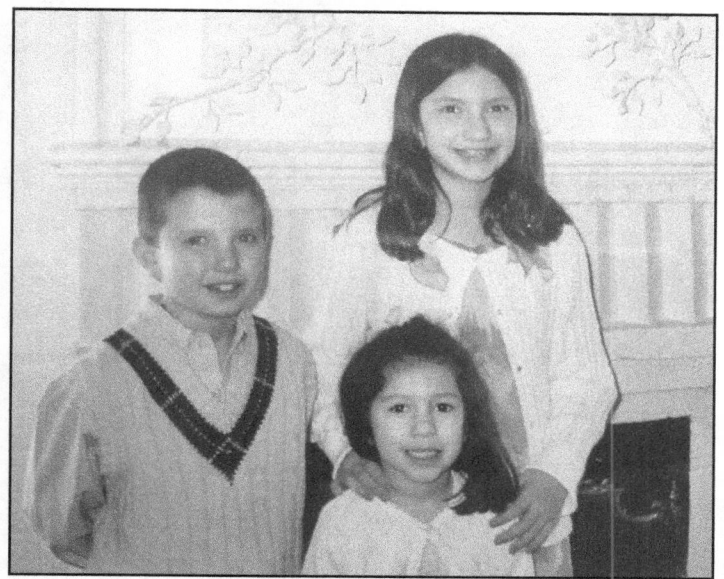

Little Eddie, Isabelle, and Sarah at their grandmother's house in Wilmette.

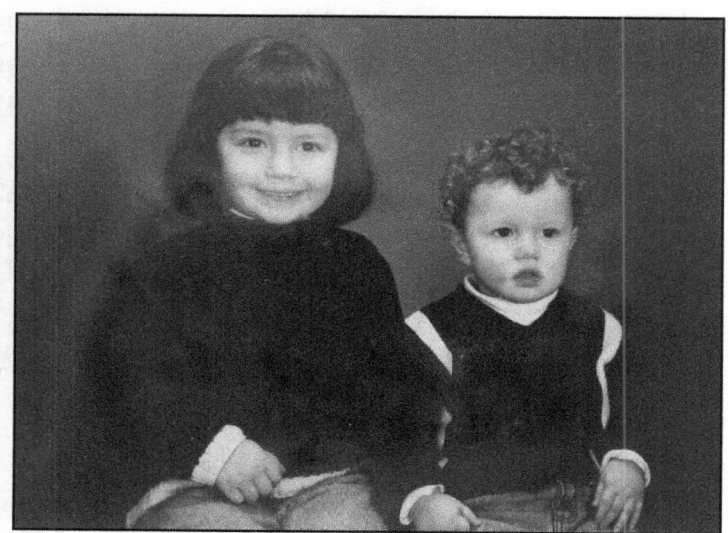

Sarah and little Eddie pose for a portrait.

DRUNK AT FIRESIDE

September 19, 1993

MY DAUGHTER, SARAH Arana, was born on September 19, 1993, in Saint Francis Hospital in Evanston, Illinois, at approximately 4 a.m. I was so happy the day she was born. She was the most remarkable creature I had ever seen. I put up a sign in the hospital room that read "Come in and see the PERFECT baby." It was a day that I will never forget. I was so proud to be her father. A lot of friends and family came to the hospital room to see Sarah and to congratulate us. It was one of the best days of my life. Anyone who has kids knows what I'm talking about.

It was about 10 p.m., and I suppose I had had enough of all the baby talk and family and friends. I told T. C. I was going to get something to eat and that I would be back in a couple of hours. I drove directly to the Fireside, a local neighborhood bar/restaurant on the North Side of Chicago near Ravenswood and Rosehill by Rosehill Cemetery (which, ironically, was previously the site of a major drunken car crash I had been involved in years earlier). I proceeded to have some scotch and some Miller Lites with a few shots of Jack Daniel's peppered in. People at the bar were buying me drinks, "congratulating" me on my great accomplishment of fathering a child. I accepted every one of those "congratulations"—one ounce at a time. The bar closed at 2 a.m., and I was bombed. I recall urinating in the bathroom at Fireside and looking in the mirror (a familiar, recurring scene) and thinking to myself, What the fuck am I doing? Why the fuck am I doing this? This shit ain't normal. Why aren't I with my family who I love so much? That thought quickly goes away though—every time. You want that thought to go away. The guilt is talking to you, and you don't want to hear about it. Deep down inside, you know what you're doing is fucked up, but you don't care. You just keep on doing it. The alcoholism wins almost every time. The alcoholism is like Vegas—it is hard to beat the house odds.

I jumped into my car so I could get home and go to sleep and make it back to the hospital without T. C. finding out that I had been drinking. Well, next thing I remember, I was still on Ravenswood, the street that Fireside was on, with the engine running. It was 5:30 a.m. A friend of mine, who was a Chicago police officer at the time, was knocking on my windshield and yelling for me to wake up. I awoke and thanked him. He congratulated me for Sarah, and I was on my merry way. I eventually went to the hospital to see how Sarah and T. C. were doing. They were doing just fine. I had gotten away scot-free with another drinking near-miss! Aren't I wonderful, Sarah? Don't you have a great Dad? Don't you want to grow up with a father who has these types of morals? Don't you want a father who would leave his daughter the day she was born just so he could get fucked up? My daughter had just been born hours earlier, and I chose my alcoholism over her. It seems so unfathomable to me right now, but when you are in your disease, it just seems extremely normal.

The crazy shit I did in order to drink just makes me want to apologize to all those whom I had hurt—especially my children. It just wasn't worth it. I made so many stupid fucking mistakes that I now regret. The regret and guilt is almost too overwhelming at times. I cannot imagine what would have happened if I had continued to drink. I am sure I would be dead by now. Sobriety lets you right a lot of wrongs in life. If Sarah ever has a baby, I will be the first one in that hospital room, and I will be the last one to leave. I have my sobriety to thank for that type of thinking now.

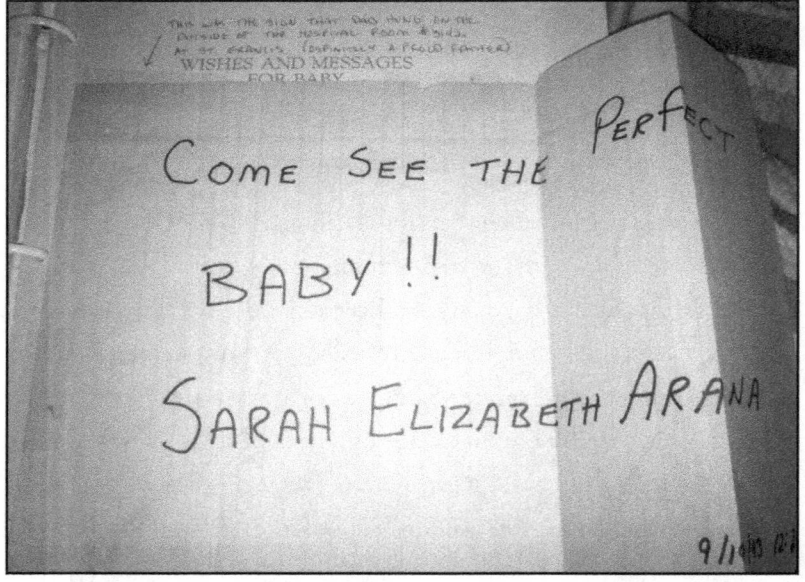

A picture of the note I left outside the hospital room when Sarah was born.

EATIN'S CHEATIN'

July 21, 1999

STEVE BREWER WAS one of my main drinking partners during my heyday. He loved to drink Grey Goose vodka—straight with only ice. I really looked up to him as a drinking legend. He had the very dangerous combination of a desire to drink a lot and often and a seemingly endless bank account. He was a real pleasure to drink with. He seemed to appreciate alcohol as much as I did. It was like he didn't take it for granted. I admired that quality in a person. Steve could drink a lot more than I could. He was a bigger, muscular guy, so it took a lot more alcohol in his system to get him fucked up. I am a short, fat, ugly Peruvian man. It did not take that much for me to get fucked up.

Steve Brewer adhered to many of the same drinking "rules" that I did. A drinking "rule" is an unspoken guideline among drinkers. For example, if someone offers you a shot of any kind, you never say no—you just drink it like a man, no matter how you feel or how drunk you are in the moment. It was a drinker's omertà of sorts, a code of silence that all-star drinkers used when asked if they were drunk or not. They never admitted it and were always ready for another drink. I really admired that type of shit. Another "rule" that Steve constantly harped on was called "eatin's cheatin'"—which meant that you could not eat while you drank because the food would ruin the effect of the alcohol, effectively "cheating" you of the buzz you had worked so hard to get. So, Steve frowned upon the eating of any food while we were on our drinking binges. If a waitress asked us if we wanted anything to eat while we were at a bar or restaurant, Steve would always reply with his patented line: "Nope, eatin's cheatin.'" I never ate and mainly drank because I hated the taste of alcohol and I loved the taste of food—and I didn't want the alcohol to ruin my meal.

Steve and I attended a Cubs game on a warm and sunny Wednesday afternoon in Chicago. We met at Bernie's, a bar located directly across the street from Wrigley Field. We met at the standard 11:30 a.m. starting time, which was approximately two hours prior to the scheduled first pitch. We knew all of the bartenders at Bernie's, so even in a packed bar, we got our drinks very quickly. Steve drank his Grey Goose on the rocks, and I drank Miller Lite. We each had approximately six to eight drinks before we left Bernie's to enter Wrigley Field in the third inning. We sat down at our seats in Club Box section 26 row 6, which was six rows from the field directly behind the visitors on-deck circle. Great seats for base-ball, but more importantly, great seats for drinking. Beer was the only option to drink at Wrigley Field at the time unless you were a member of the Stadium Club, where you could get mixed drinks. Steve and I ordered four beers at a time per inning up until the seventh inning stretch—that would be about twenty beers total (ten beers each). We left the ballpark around the eighth inning. Please don't ask who the Cubs were playing or what the score was or if the Cubs had won or not, because I have zero recollection. Things get very fuzzy at this point. Steve had mentioned that he wanted to go to Yak-Zies, which was another bar on Clark Street across the street from Wrigley Field. I needed to go to the bathroom, and I told him I would meet him at Yak-Zies after I urinated.

After I went to the bathroom at Wrigley Field, I went to look for Brewer at Yak-Zies. He was nowhere to be found. I even ordered a couple of Miller Lites and a shot just to get my head together. I asked the bartender if he had seen Steve, and he said he had seen him earlier but that he had left. Now, I was getting worried. Where the fuck was Brewer? I hated drinking by myself! Where was my running partner?

I left Yak-Zies and went down the block back to Bernie's. I asked Brian, the only Asian bartender in Chicago with an Italian accent, if he had seen Brewer. He said he had seen him about a half hour earlier because he had ordered a Grey Goose on the rocks. I went toward the back of Bernie's where there was a large tent-like structure set up with a grill that they used to prepare food. I knew he wouldn't be there because we did not eat while we drank. I looked and looked around— still no sign of Brewer. I had to urinate again, so I went inside the bathroom. There were only two toilet stalls at Bernie's. One of those stalls was occupied, and upon closer inspection, I noticed a familiar pair of expensive shoes protruding under the door. It was Brewer! I had found him. It was very loud outside the bathroom but eerily quiet inside. I wondered what the fuck this guy was doing. Had he fallen asleep? Had he passed out? Was he even alive? I quickly opened the door of the bathroom stall, and I witnessed a scene that will forever remain etched in my mind: there was Brewer with the biggest shit-eating grin you could ever see on a human being, holding a gigantic double cheeseburger with everything on it from the grill (prepared by Bernie's master chef, Javier, no doubt). This motherfucker was eating! And this motherfucker was trying to hide it from me! And he was eating like his next stop was the electric chair.

Eatin's cheatin', huh, Steve?

You motherfucker!

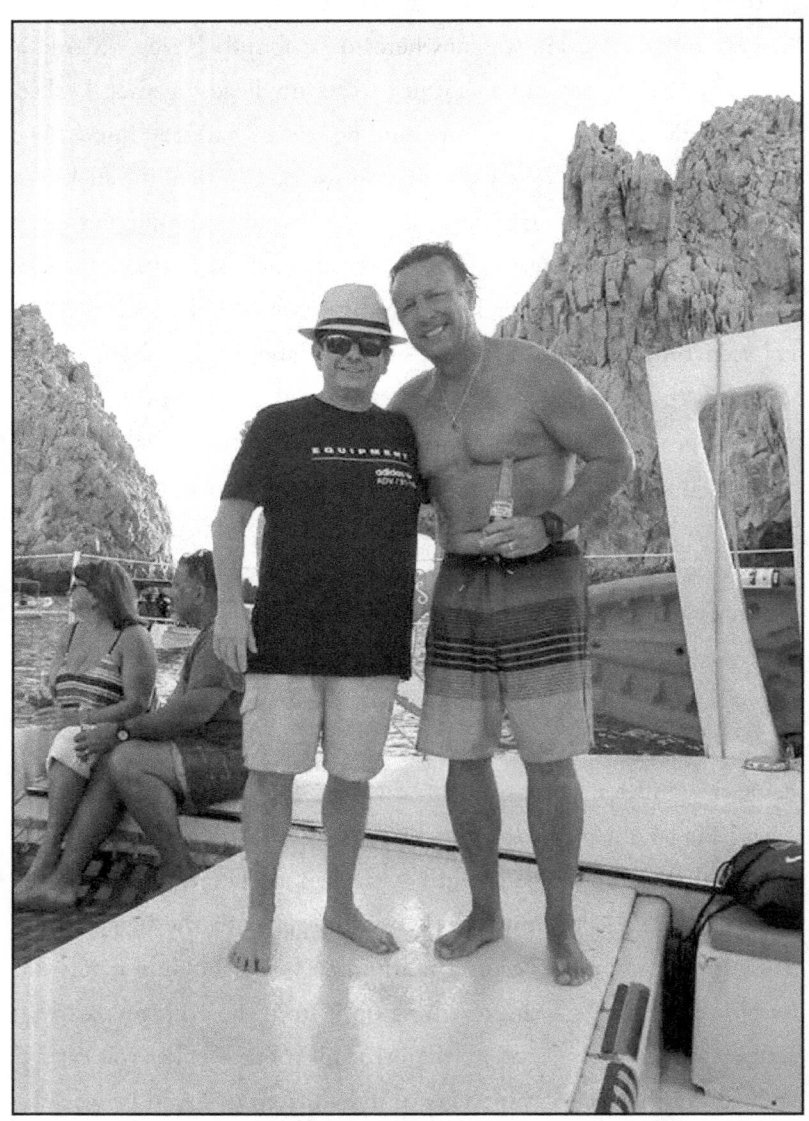

Steve Brewer and I in Cabo San Lucas, January 2018.

FIRST PIANO RECITAL

July 2000

THIS PARTICULAR DRINKING story affects me more than any other story. So many things went wrong, and they were all avoidable. The day started off innocently enough. I was invited to the Western Open golf tournament at the Medinah Country Club in Medinah, Illinois, which was about forty-five minutes from where I lived. It was a "work outing" on a Thursday. I received a ride to the tournament from a work friend because I did not want to drink and drive. Before I left, T. C. asked me to be home by 6:30 p.m. because Sarah, my oldest daughter who was seven at the time, was going to have her first piano recital that night at a church in Park Ridge, about five minutes from our house. She had been taking lessons and practicing the piano for about two years. This was a big deal to her. I didn't think getting home by 6:30 p.m. would be a problem.

We left for the golf tournament around 7 a.m. We arrived at 8 a.m. and went straight to the hospitality tent, which was basically an open bar with many TV sets covering the tournament. I was drinking single malt scotch, Glenlivet. I drank the entire day. I must have had at least twenty drinks. They had real glasses at this event as opposed to plastic cups. It is amazing the details that one recalls about certain events even if you are fucked up beyond all recognition. The acronym that kids use these days for this condition is known as FUBAR'd (Fucked Up Beyond All Recognition). I also did a few shots of Jack Daniel's.

Twenty drinks are a lot for one person to handle. I supposed I could handle my alcohol pretty well—or so I thought. I never left the hospitality tent the entire day—10 hours. I averaged about two drinks an hour, which doesn't really sound too bad when you look at it on an hourly basis (a famous trick that drunks use so as not to appear that they drink excessively). I kept looking at the clock, thinking to myself: I gotta be home by 6:30 p.m. or T. C. is going to kill me. But, those single malt scotches kept coming and coming. I was on a roll, and I had to go to this fucking piano recital. What the fuck! Okay, now it was about 5:30 p.m, and my work friends were all aware that I needed to get home. So, naturally, I ordered one final Glenlivet. "Make this one a double, bartender!"

Drunks like to ensure that they can keep their buzz going when they know they will be entering an alcohol-free environment: for example, a church in Park Ridge to witness a piano recital. When it was 6:30 p.m., I was still at the Medinah Country Club. I was obviously not going to make it home by 6:30. I called T. C. and told her that I had gotten "held up" at the tournament with "work stuff" and that I would just meet everyone at the church. If you are a drunk and you have a white-collar job, it is very easy to use your job as an excuse to continue to get fucked up well into the night. I called a cab (a "cab" is a vehicle that takes you to your desired location where you reach into your pocket and pay cash to the driver after the ride is over; Uber was nonexistent back then).

I made it to the church in Park Ridge by 7:25 p.m. I had made it! I had not disappointed my daughter. I was a hero! My whole family was there—my mom, my dad, my two other kids, and my in-laws. Everyone was present to see little Sarah's first piano recital. I realized that I was very fucked up, so I didn't want to sit with everyone in the front. My family had gotten there early to reserve the seats in the first two rows of the church. Thank god the church had a balcony upstairs. I decided to go up there for a while before Sarah performed just so I could buy a little time and let some of the fucking scotch wear off. I was really fucked up.

The next memory is rather fuzzy. I remember being shaken by a woman whom I did not know and being asked to leave the church. Apparently, I had been snoring so loudly that it was affecting the performances. I was escorted out of the building. Everyone witnessed it, including my daughter Sarah. I missed her entire performance that evening. I woke up on a park bench near the church and walked home at 10 p.m.

At the time, I did not really consider this incident a big deal. I mean, I went to the fucking recital; I just missed her part because I had fallen asleep. The more time that passes, the bigger of a deal that night becomes for me. Imagine being an innocent, little seven-year-old girl who is so excited about her first performance. She had been practicing and taking lessons for two years. Her entire family is there. And then her dad, the town fucking drunk, passes out upstairs and is asked to leave. What the fuck must she have thought? She was seven years old and my oldest daughter. What kind of a fucking monster was I?

I have apologized many times to Sarah about that night. I feel horrible about what happened. The only way I can make this thing right is by attending Sarah's daughter's or son's (if she has kids) first piano recital. I promise I will get there early, and I promise to sit up front. I promise that I will be sober, and I promise never to embarrass her again. Sarah, I love you with all of my heart; and I apologize, again, for that night.

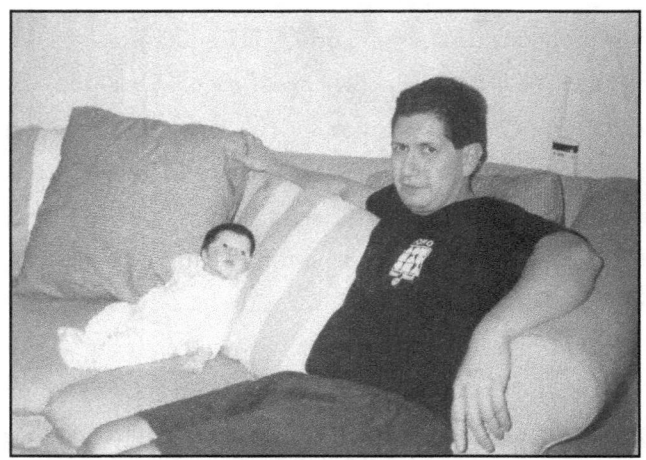

Sarah staring at me in amazement. I wonder what she was thinking?

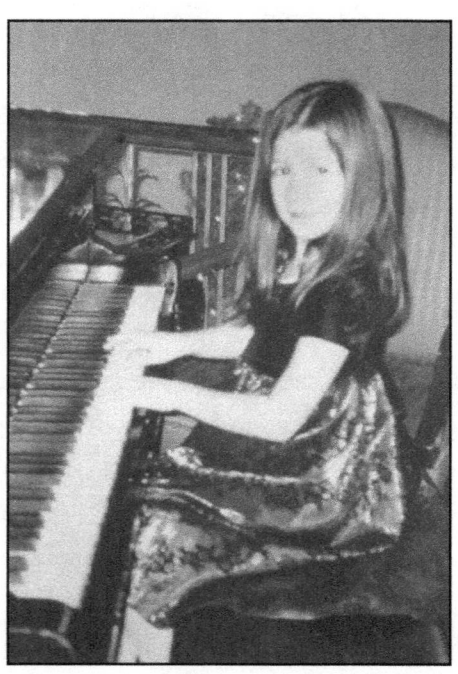

Isabelle playing the piano. She looks just like Sarah in this picture.

JACK WALSH: BOB

June 2001

JACK WALSH INTRODUCED me to single malt scotch, Glenlivet to be exact. Jack Walsh also participated in an incident that was the beginning of the end of my marriage. I used to work with Jack at a German bank called Commerzbank. He was the vice president of sales and I was the chief financial officer. I could never understand a fucking word the guy used in normal conversations. He was very intelligent. He used big words. Many of my afternoons would be spent in his office drinking scotch and talking about life. It was mostly Jack talking and me understanding about one-eighth of what he said. We would have contests in the office to determine if a certain word he had used actually existed. After being fact-checked, every word was legitimate, by the way.

Jack Walsh was a gentleman. He got into an altercation one morning in Downtown Chicago, right in the middle of Wacker Drive near the Sears Tower. Jack had a quick temper and felt that the man had somehow disrespected him as he was walking across the street. He squared off against this man, who was at least thirty years his junior and in much better shape. Jack positioned himself in the classic, old school John L. Sullivan boxer's stance. At this point there were about fifty people witnessing this spectacle, including myself. The fight was a two-hit fight. The guy hit Jack, and Jack hit the ground. Jack got up and realized he had blood all over his shirt. He hailed a cab and instructed the driver in a very gentlemanly fashion, "Driver, please take me to Brooks Brothers. I must purchase a new shirt."

Jack and I went out drinking one night. Jack loved to drink, and so the fuck did I. We were perfect for each other. Jack had an older car that he affectionately named BOB, which stood for "Bucket of Bolts." We had gone to several downtown taverns and enjoyed our favorite drink, Glenlivet, at each one of those bars. It was about 2 a.m., and Jack announced that he had had enough to drink. He offered to drive me home. I was equally as drunk as Jack, but he was a much more seasoned drinker than I was at the time. Jack did not even live near me, but this was the kind of guy Jack was, and I am sure continues to be.

I lived in Park Ridge, a nice little community near Chicago's Northwest Side. We were coming from downtown, which is about a twenty-minute drive. At the time, T.C. was doing a major reconstruction to our home. She was building an addition to the back of the house, and there were all kinds of construction going on in the backyard. Jack and I arrived at my house at about 2:30 a.m. I thanked Jack for the ride and told him I would just get out of BOB. Jack, however, insisted and announced, "I am a gentleman. I will pull up to your driveway and drop you off properly." I had completely forgotten that the construction crew had dug a hole in the backyard about thirty feet deep. It was very dark outside, and before you know it, old Bucket of Bolts had fallen into this gaping hole with me and Jack in the car. I remember a loud thud and realized what had happened. In retrospect, Jack must have pressed on the gas pedal because we fell perfectly into the hole. We did not know what to do.

The next morning, I remember T. C. screaming at Jack and I to get out of the car and to get out of the hole. I was actually hugging Jack, and I guess we had fallen asleep in that position for a few hours. T. C. just walked around the hole, shaking her head, and left for work as if what she had just witnessed was perfectly normal. Eventually, the construction men arrived and pulled BOB, Jack, and myself out of the hole with a crane. I think it was safe to say that this was the beginning of the end of my marriage. Can you imagine what the neighbors thought when they saw two grown men hugging each other in a car that had fallen in a hole in our backyard?

T. C. continues to deny that this incident ever took place. I can imagine that as a wife and a mother to our three children, it is extremely embarrassing to admit that she would have allowed behavior like this to take place. I am not proud of what happened that night. However, I do see the humor in it. I understand that T. C. would love to wipe this memory from her brain. If I was married to someone who continually behaved in this manner, I do not believe I would have lasted long in the marriage, either. This was one of those "legendary" stories that I was so eager to have in my drinking arsenal. Now, it just seems so ridiculous. Why would I put my wife and my kids through this type of thing? They all deserved better.

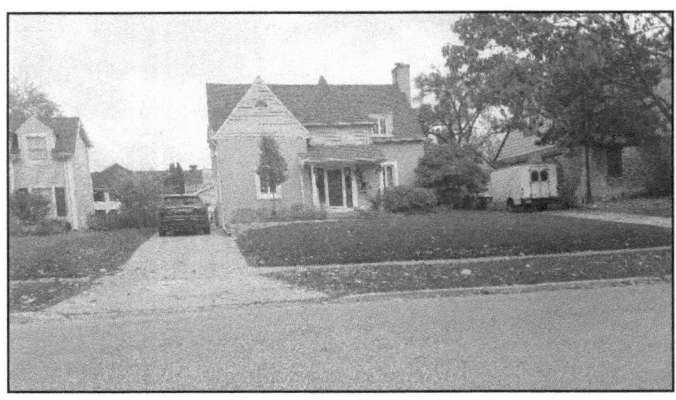

This was our house in Park Ridge—notice the long driveway where Jack and I drove into a hole.

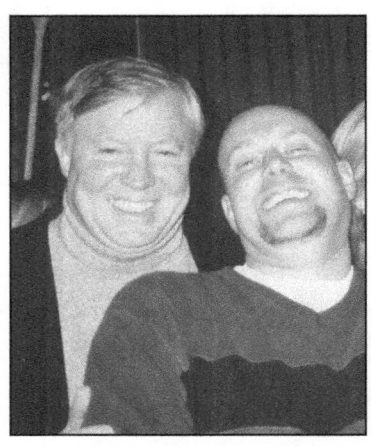

Jack Walsh and Jimmy Piske in the year 2000. Jack and Jimmy were major influences in my drinking life. I love both of these guys.

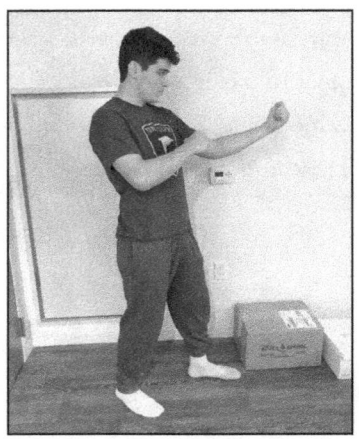

The John L. Sullivan boxing pose.

TAKING THE GARBAGE OUT

July 2001

"I AM NOT joining a fucking country club."

T. C. and I had just joined the Park Ridge Country Club. I had never wanted to join because I did not have any interest in being a member of a country club. I thought it was pretentious and that all of the people who belonged to one were snobby. Joining the club was a concession that I had to make to my wife in order to keep her happy. I had a very limited amount of friends who were members, and I did not look forward to attending any events.

It was a Wednesday night, and I was taking out the garbage. The garbage cans had to be put out on the street for the garbage men to pick up on Thursday morning. As I was setting the garbage cans down, I saw two friends of mine driving down the street. They stopped and asked me if I wanted to stop by the 19th Hole, a bar and lounge area at the Park Ridge Country Club where men relax, and have a drink and play Ship, Captain, Crew. I knew how to drink but I had no fucking idea what Ship, Captain, Crew was.

We lived about a block and a half from the country club. I decided to see what it was all about. I walked over at about 9 p.m., and it was paradise. There were about fifteen guys at the 19th Hole drinking scotch, playing cards, watching sports on television, eating pizza, and telling insensitive jokes. This was nirvana to me. I had hit the fucking jackpot!

Apparently, Ship, Captain, Crew was a dice game. Within an hour, I had lost $1,200 playing that ridiculous game. Nobody at the club seemed to be affected by losing that kind of money. Growing up, I used to watch my dad and his friends play a dice game that involved dice and a cup. I learned how to do several tricks with the dice, flipping the cup into the air while the dice were still in it. My skills with the dice cup fascinated my newfound friends. Thankfully, the scotches just kept flowing, and I forgot about the money that I had just lost. It was now about 2 a.m. I was no longer playing Ship, Captain, Crew. I was just drinking. Sammy the bartender made a great scotch on the rocks. A few of us decided to go to Rivers Casino to gamble some more. I didn't gamble, but I sure drank. Glenlivet was going down like water. We stayed at the casino until 4 a.m. or so, and then we decided to get something to eat. We went to an all-night diner and ate some steak and eggs. It was delicious—I think.

By now, it was about 7 a.m., and we went back to the 19th Hole to play some more Ship, Captain, Crew. I believe I won some of my money back. However, I do remember continuing my drinking of single malt scotch. We drank the entire day. There were several groups of guys who came in after their rounds of golf. I did not play golf, but I made so many new friends that day. I was known as the new member who drank and never went home. I had lunch at the 19th Hole and continued to drink. Keep in mind that it was now Thursday afternoon. My wife had been calling nonstop, and I was not answering the phone. She thought I had just left the house to take out the garbage, and she had no idea where I had gone.

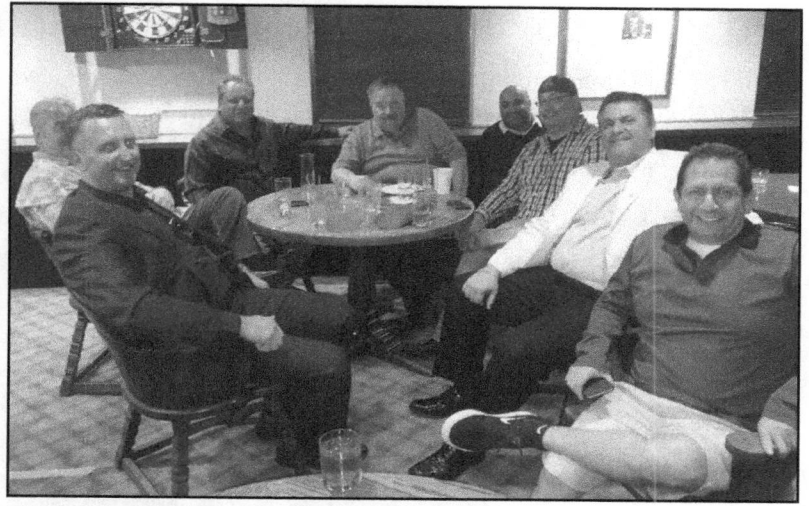

The infamous 19th Hole at the Park Ridge Country Club
(pictured from left to right: George Tolczyk, Matt Pilolli, Joe Petrecca,
Freddie Kunzer, Axay Gandhi, Steve Cueto, Angelo Demeros and myself.)

Why the fuck should I answer her calls? I thought. She had made me join this fucking club. I was making the best of it. There are moments like this when you instinctively know what you have to do, and yet you just do not do it. I just kept burying myself deeper and deeper into this nineteenth hole (pun intended).

It was now Thursday night, and I was *still* drinking and trying to play Ship, Captain, Crew. I passed out on a chair in the 19th Hole and woke up around 3 a.m. There were still guys playing the game. This was the country club for me! I had made some great new friends that day. I was sure T. C. was ecstatic to know that I had fit right in with the country club crowd. I walked home and went right to bed. T. C. was very angry with me.

I thought to myself, Big fucking deal. I had fun.

I have told this story many times to the guys at the Park Ridge Country Club. Everyone thinks it is hilarious. The story has attained legendary status, which was all I ever wanted in life. My popularity was always based on something outrageous that I had done while drinking. I could not have asked for more. It was a great story—or so I thought.

The thing that wasn't so funny was that I had a wife and kids who were worried sick about me. I could have been dead somewhere—but I didn't give a fuck. All I cared about was me and making sure that I had fun. I wanted the story to be good; I wanted to have the best stories so I could laugh about them later. It was like I was creating content so people could talk about me.

This was a pattern I would follow for the rest of my life—even into sobriety.

THE CUPCAKE

October 2001

MY OLDEST DAUGHTER, Sarah, has always been scared of costumes. As an infant, she was terrified of Halloween or any holiday involving costumes—or anything remotely resembling a costume for that matter. On her second birthday in 1995, I dressed up in a Cookie Monster costume and scared the Peruvian out of her. I was so drunk that I passed out in the alley behind our house in this costume. She had seen the Cookie Monster laying there, lifeless. I am sure this incident didn't help her through her fear of costumes. There is no rhyme or reason for this fear; she simply has it.

Let us fast forward to the year 2001. Sarah was eight years old. Sarah was eight years old. Sarah was eight years old. That is not a typo. I want everyone to know what a fucked up thing I did to an eight-year-old girl—and, to make matters worse, my own daughter. My old high school, Gordon Tech, was playing a big playoff game (basketball) that night. Some of my old crew were going to meet there, and then we were going to decide where to go get drunk after the game. I hadn't seen a lot of these guys in years, so I was really looking forward to the game and seeing all my friends whose names all escape me right now (that is how important they really were to me). Sarah and I walked into the gym. We had to wait in a long line to get in. The place was packed to the rafters, and there was a wonderful high-school-basketball vibe in the air. Sarah was hungry, so I purchased her a nice little chocolate cupcake with strawberry frosting on it. She was very happy and saved it so she could eat it during the game.

My buddies had reserved us a couple of spots in the bleachers at the far end of the gym. As we entered the GT gym, there he was—the Gordon Tech Ram mascot (cue the eerily scary music). Sarah went absolutely ballistic. She could not walk any farther into the gym. I really thought that at her age, her fear of these costumes was over and that she could overcome it. She started bawling uncontrollably and refused to step one foot into the gym. I yelled, "What the fuck, Sarah? It's only a fucking costume!" My yelling and tone made her cry even harder. I had no choice but to take her home. I was so fucking pissed. I didn't get a chance to see my friends or to find out where the fuck we were going after the game to get fucked up. Could you believe that fucking daughter of mine? She had a lot of fucking nerve to start crying and fuck up my good time! Damn right I was pissed, and for good reason. As we were walking to the parking lot, I yelled at her, "Give me that fucking cupcake!" She handed me the uneaten cupcake, and I threw it as far as I could onto California Avenue. Fuck that shit. We drove home and didn't say a word. The crying had stopped only because the costumes were no longer there. I vowed in my mind to never take her to another sporting event again.

Well. I guess it takes many years to fully understand what I did that night. I yelled at the person who was the most precious thing to me in my entire life—the "perfect baby" as I had described her the day she was born. I yelled and ranted and raved because I had wanted to get fucked up and she prevented me from doing so. Today, Sarah and I talk about this incident a lot and kind of laugh about it as a funny thing. But, fuck, years later, it ain't so funny. I am truly sorry, Sarah, for doing that to you that night. You have no idea of the regret that I have for treating you like that. You were only eight years old, a little kid who was scared. I just wanted to get fucked up so badly. Now, I don't get fucked up anymore.

I WILL NEVER DO THAT TO YOU AGAIN.

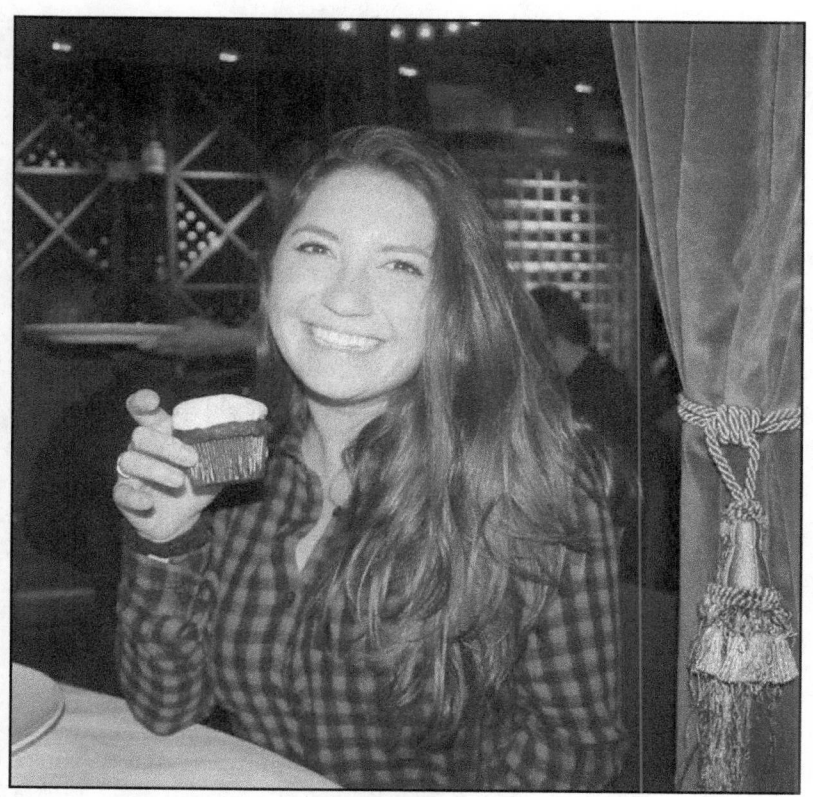

This is my daughter, Sarah, who claims she has gotten over "the cupcake" incident.

FRANK DIFRANCO

July 2004

"YOU GOTTA CALL Frank."

I was lying in a hospital bed on July 15, 2004 around 5 a.m. at Lutheran General Hospital in Park Ridge and had just woken up. "How the fuck did I get here?" My face was all bruised and cut up. My entire body was shaking. I was strapped to my bed in a straitjacket.

I called my friend Jimmy Roppel, local celebrity hedge fund manager, for advice; I had been charged with a DUI, and I was in major trouble. I need legal assistance. The only thing that came out of his mouth was better than any financial advice he would ever give his clients. He said, "You gotta call Frank." I bet if I trademarked the saying "You gotta call Frank," I would be retired right now with multiple houses in Park Ridge alone. He was referring to Frank DiFranco of DiFranco and Associates, an attorney with a practice in Park Ridge, Illinois. Jimmy gave me Frank's number, and I called him that morning from my hospital bed. Frank gave me his home address and told me to go straight to his house to talk when I was released.

When Frank speaks, you listen and you comply. I arrived at Frank's house looking like hell. My head and face were bandaged up and I had bloodstains all over my clothes. Frank's wife, Angela, made me a delicious turkey sandwich with potato chips. Again, the details that you remember while you are drunk or coming off of a drunken night are remarkable. It was the best turkey sandwich I had ever eaten in my life. We discussed what happened that evening, and Frank told me, "Don't worry about it, buddy. Everything is going to be okay."

Well, everything was not okay. I had been involved in a major car accident, and my whole life was falling apart. As I was leaving, Frank also threw out there: "Hey buddy, it might be a good idea to go to one of those AA meetings. I know you don't have a problem or anything like that, but it looks good to the court system if they see you are taking steps to make sure this never happens again."

"Thanks a lot, Frank."

A few days later, Roppel called me and asked if I had spoken to Frank. I told him that I had. Jimmy then said, "Do exactly what Frank tells you to do."

That evening, I went to my very first AA meeting on Busse Highway at the Maine Center in Park Ridge (the details of that first AA meeting are covered in a later chapter). However, prior to that, I had already known for a long time that I was an alcoholic. I believe any alcoholic is fully aware of their problem way before they actually do anything about it. Going to an AA meeting was a major fear for me. I knew that I would be exposed. I was very cognizant of what would come out at that meeting—and that terrified me. I hate change, and this would turn my entire life upside down—and I wanted no part of it. However, I had been told to listen to Frank DiFranco. He was an expert in this business.

The night before the meeting, I was still considering not going. I was trying to figure out if there was any other way I could somehow make amends or pay a fine or take a class—anything but an AA meeting. But those words from Roppel kept ringing in my head:

"Do exactly what Frank tells you to do."

For the first time, I want to publicly thank Frank DiFranco. He had known fully well that I had a major problem, and he had advised me in a way that did not embarrass me. He treated me like a human being, not like the degenerate drunk I was. I really owe a great deal of gratitude to Frank for that fantastic piece of advice he had given me—to go to an AA meeting. Sometimes, it takes some pushing to do the thing you already know you have to do but that you just cannot bring yourself to do. It seemed like such an obvious thing to say to someone—go to an AA meeting—but if it had been said offensively or with a judgmental tone, it would not have resonated with me.

Thank you, buddy. You saved my life. I did exactly what you told me to do.

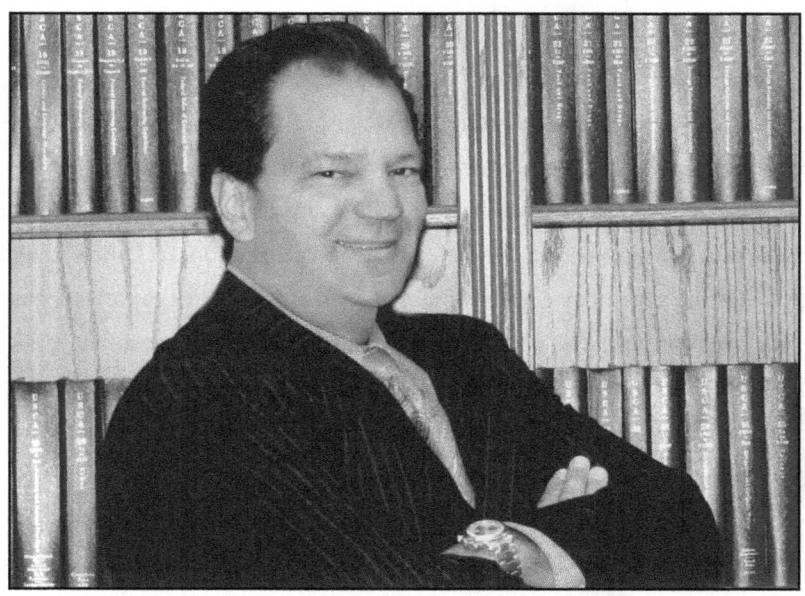

Frank DiFranco, one of the top defense lawyers in the country.

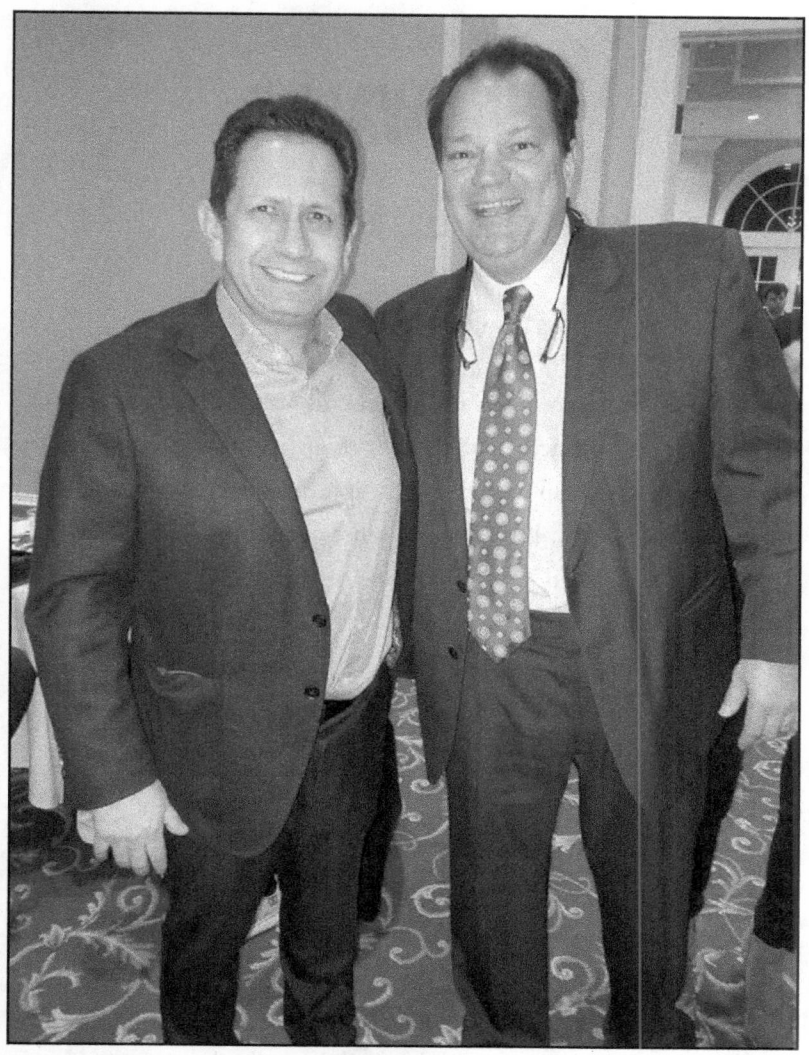

Frank DiFranco and I at a fundraiser when Frank ran for judge in 2020.

THE "WALK"

July 22, 2004

T. C. AND I decided to take a neighborhood walk in Park Ridge about a week after my car accident. Besides receiving stitches and assorted bumps and bruises (and a DUI), my injuries were minor, and I felt pretty good physically. I felt a major sense of relief—like I had dodged another bullet. I asked T. C. if she wanted to go to Zia's, which is an Italian restaurant in the neighboring town of Edison Park. I also asked her if she wouldn't mind if I had one beer so we could "celebrate" me getting out of the hospital and getting our lives "back to normal."

Let's rewind:

When T. C. first arrived at the hospital the week before and I was lying down strapped to the hospital bed, she told me in no uncertain terms:

"Eddie, if you have *one* more drink, I will divorce you."

I really did not think she was serious. I did not think this incident was more serious than the past situations I had put myself and my family in. She had threatened me plenty of times, and nothing had really come out of her threats. I figured she would eventually feel sorry for me

128

and not be too angry—and that we could continue on with our lives. What was one beer? Would it hurt? The worst was behind us; I just had to be more careful about drinking and driving. What was the big deal? T. C. had known who I was when she married me, I thought. I didn't really plan on changing. This was not a part of my life that I wanted to change, no fucking way. I was not going to take away one of the only enjoyable things I thought I had in my life. Yes, I had had a few close calls, but I was good now, and I was getting healthy, and everything was going to be okay, right? Let's go to Zia's and celebrate with one little beer, okay?

T. C.'s reaction (and I remember this reaction like it happened five minutes ago):

"Eddie, I told you that if you have one more drink, I will divorce you. I am serious. Don't fuck with me."

This was not the reaction I had been hoping for. This was a reaction of a person who was as serious as a heart attack. Usually, I would have tried to press it and convince her that this would not be a big deal. But something in the tone of her voice made me believe that she was not fucking around. I knew that T. C. was not going to budge this time. I saw the pain in her eyes. She did not want any more incidents. She did not want any more embarrassing moments regarding her husband. She did not want her kids to have a father whom people laughed at and did not take seriously. It was a big moment for me. T. C. had said she was going to divorce me.

Holy fuck! I couldn't believe this was happening to me. I could not have that. Peruvians do not get divorced. They work it out no matter what happens. Naively, I thought: I am going to have to figure out a way to continue to drink and to keep her happy. How was I going to do this? She was so fucking mad at me, and she was serious this time.

Not drinking at all was 100 percent out of the question. Drinking was a huge part of my life. Most, if not all, of my human social interactions were based on alcohol. This was a major problem. How was I going to fix this? I was really going to have to think about this one.

The mind of an alcoholic is very direct and focused. I had to figure out a way to hold on to my marriage, yet continue to drink as much as I wanted and whenever I wanted to. It was very depressing to think about a life without my alcohol.

THINK, EDDIE, THINK.

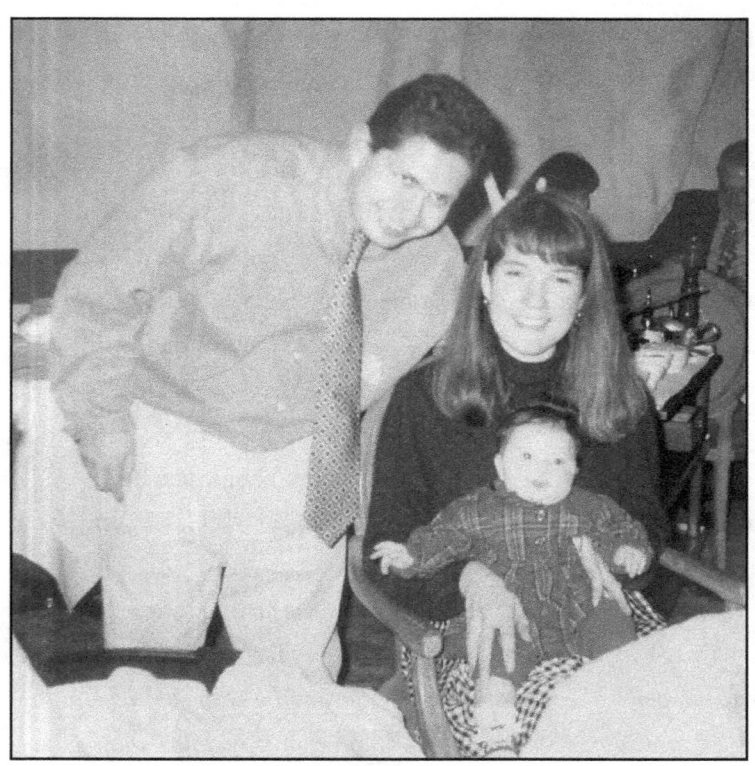

Me, T. C., and Sarah at Café Le Cave restaurant in Rosemont, Illinois.

MY FIRST AA (ALCOHOLICS ANONYMOUS) MEETING

July 2004

THE ONLY REASON I went to my first AA meeting was because I wanted people to think that I was doing something about my drinking. My lawyer Frank DiFranco had suggested I go to the meeting prior to my court case. I had gotten into a major car accident, totaled my car and damaged city property, been charged with a DUI, been suspended from the country club, and was getting alienated from my wife and kids—all from one night of drinking.

The first AA meeting I attended was a nightmare come true. When I arrived, I was extremely nervous. I had to admit to everyone that I was an alcoholic. The secret was going to come out. I had tried so hard for so many years to hide it and pretend like I was normal. But deep down, I knew it was time. I could not even begin to describe the number of incidents that had happened to me because of my drinking. Overwhelming guilt due to my drinking and the effect it had on my family and friends overcame me that night. It was horrible.

There were people at the meeting from all ages ranging from seventeen to seventy-five years old. I thought: What am I doing here with these fucking losers, and how did it get so bad that I am actually here? There were people present who were not dressed properly and who looked like they had just crawled out from underneath a rock. I pulled into the place in a fucking Mercedes. There were people there on bicycles and people who had come off the bus. There were toothless women who looked like they had just been hit by a train—it was not exactly a good place to pick up women. I was so much better than this. I was a member of the Park Ridge Country Club, for god's sake. When was this fucking thing going to be over?

The main person leading the session asked if this was anyone's first AA meeting. Nobody raised their hand. There was no way that I was going to announce to these people that this was my first time. It was so embarrassing. I did not know the protocol of the meeting, so I just remained silent and still. I was counting the seconds till this thing was going to end.

Typically, the first half hour of an AA meeting is spent reading AA book passages, usually one of the twelve steps. That was easy enough. Everyone sat on a couch in a circle. People took turns reading different paragraphs from the books. I considered myself a pretty good reader, so when it came my turn to read, I felt like I dominated the reading portion. Some of the people had a hard time reading. I felt so foolishly superior to them. I wanted them to hurry up and finish the paragraph so we could get on to the next reader. In hindsight, this was a big part of my problem all along. I knew I had a major problem, and when anyone tried to address it with me, I would just speed things along and pretend like it never happened.

The second half of the hour was the hard part—the talking part. The leader of the meeting went around the room and asked us to speak about what we had thought of the reading or anything else that was on our minds. Seven people spoke until it became my turn. Every one of those seven people had started their speech with the following: "My name is so-and-so, and I am an alcoholic."

The people who spoke ahead of me mentioned that drinking had caused them to lose everything in their lives. Someone spoke about having had to travel to that meeting on a bus and almost missing the bus. Someone spoke about how drinking had caused friction among their family members. Some of their stories resonated with me, while some were laughable. Remember, I did not want to admit anything to anyone at this point.

Now I had a decision to make. Thoughts raced through my mind. Do I introduce myself as an alcoholic even though I don't want anyone to know? Do I just pass on speaking? Do I just introduce myself and say that I am only going to listen? What the fuck should I do? Why had I even come to attend this nonsense? This is such a complete waste of my time.

When it came to my turn to speak, I quickly announced, "Hi, my name is Eddie, and I'm an alcoholic." It was extremely hard for me to get those words out. "I am an alcoholic," "I am an alcoholic," "I am an alcoholic." I couldn't believe I was actually saying it. I fucking said that I was an alcoholic! I never really believed it until I said those words out loud at that meeting. It was a very strange thing to say. It felt like the weight of the world had been lifted from my shoulders. For the majority of my life, I had known that there was something very wrong with me, yet I had refused to admit it. The AA meeting was the perfect opportunity to release those emotions. Everyone else there was admitting that they were an alcoholic, and I was not out of place.

The gig was up.

I told my story that night. I told everyone how I had been involved in a horrible car accident and had almost died. I told everyone that I had a fantastic family and three kids but it never stopped me from drinking. I told everyone that I wanted to stop and that I wanted help. I had to pause several times during my sharing because I could not hold back the tears. It was such an unexpected emotional moment for me—extremely powerful. I felt that it was such an honest thing for me to say. I was not used to this kind of honesty—ever.

I also admitted to the group that this was my first AA meeting. I had felt guilty about not admitting it earlier. After the meeting, a wave of people tried to talk to me with information about books, phone numbers, and meeting times. I could not wait to leave that building. I practically ran out of there. I felt a combination of relief, anxiety, and fear. I was so relieved that I had finally admitted that I was an alcoholic. But I felt anxiety and fear because I was scared of the repercussions of admitting such a thing to a group of people—and really because I was also admitting it to myself.

On my drive home, I came to the realization that I may never drink again—that sucked. Also, when I'd just gotten into my car, I turned on the radio, and the first song that played was "I Can See Clearly Now" by Johnny Nash. I had heard that song a thousand times but never paid attention to the lyrics—until then.

Holy shit! Was God speaking to me? Was this some type of sign? It was a moment I will never forget. I am a huge believer in karma and in signs. This was a huge sign in my life that I had made the right decision by going to that meeting that night.

I continued to attend that particular meeting at the Main Center on Busse Highway for about one year. It was cathartic to listen to other people's stories of how screwed up their lives had become. I felt like I was not alone that I was not that bad. There were people out there who were in way worse situations than I was. I could learn from everyone there, even in a small way.

I had become quite proficient in telling my story at these meetings, and people seemed to genuinely like me. I started bringing pizzas and burgers to the meetings. I discovered that you can become very popular when you supply others with food. Coffee is also a gigantic deal at AA meetings. I have never had a cup of coffee in my life. I suppose I replaced the coffee with pizza and burgers just to be able to "fit in" better at the meetings.

I asked the most ridiculous questions to people, and they would answer me honestly. There was no subject that was out of bounds. You learn a lot about yourself at these meetings. I just kept going and going and going. It's Wednesday night—meeting night! I was so excited for every session; I could not wait to go. After my divorce, however, I had a major dilemma. My custody time with my three kids included every Wednesday night and every other weekend. I had AA meetings on Wednesday night. What was I going to do?

Fuck it. I had to take the kids to the AA meetings.

Sarah, little Eddie, and Isabelle would just sit in the corner of the room at the meetings by themselves. I have always wondered what the kids were thinking about during this time. I am sure that they just wanted to get the hell out of there and go out to eat just like other kids of divorced parents.

But I loved going to the meetings. "Keep coming back," they would all say in unison. I loved hearing the stories. Every story at an AA meeting is different. However, every story is also exactly the same. Drinking or using has fucked up your life, and you want to make your life better. I learned I was no better than anyone in there. In fact, I was worse because I had believed that I didn't belong there and I had made fun of the people who were there. I was dead wrong. I discovered that I was every bit as bad (or as good) as everyone in the room. There was no difference whatsoever. I belonged. I belonged so badly that I should have been the president of the organization. The people at those meetings bared their souls to anyone who would listen just to help them control their horrible disease.

You are so brave when you go to an AA meeting. You have done something about your problem. You'll always learn something new after every meeting. When I go to meetings now, I see myself in a lot of the people who are at those meetings—especially those who are attending a meeting for the first time. I wonder if they were thinking the same shit I was thinking in 2004?

"WHO ARE THESE LOSERS IN THIS ROOM? GET ME THE FUCK OUT OF HERE!"

NOBODY WOULD HAVE STAYED WITH ME

October 1991

T. C. AND I had three beautiful and wonderful kids—Sarah, little Eddie, and Isabelle. Our kids were our greatest accomplishment together. I do not think anyone would disagree with that statement.

T. C. was very worried how she would "come off" in this book. I think she worried that she would look stupid or foolish. Well, T. C. married a runaway train. T. C. and I eventually got divorced in 2005. The divorce was devastating to me. I did not believe in divorce, and I would have done anything to stay in the marriage. As I've mentioned, Peruvians do not believe in divorce—at least my parents did not. They believed in sticking it out for the sake of the children.

The divorce coincided with the beginning of my sobriety. As I look back to what I put that poor woman through, it is a miracle that she stayed in the marriage for as long as she did. Nobody deserved that kind of treatment. What I considered funny, she considered insulting, and rightfully so.

Can you imagine a husband of yours constantly being talked about and being known as the "town drunk"? I am sure she did not sign up

137

for this when we got married. She did not sign up to worry about me every time I went out and what time I would be home—if I came home at all.

T. C. raised our three kids and did a marvelous job. For that, I will be eternally grateful to her. Every night that I went out to drink, T. C. would be home with the kids. When it was time to do homework, it was T. C. who helped them with it. When it was time to take the kids to their scheduled events or practices or school, it was T. C. who handled it. She took care of everything until she had had enough, and I certainly do not blame her for that.

She continues to be a wonderful woman, and I have nothing but great things to say about her. I embarrassed the fuck out of her, and for that I feel horrible. She never bad-mouthed me to any of her friends or family even if she had every reason to do so. Our marriage was not perfect. However, I was the one who fucked up my marriage—period. There were no excuses for my behavior other than the fact that I was an alcoholic.

The alcoholic tries to find so many different excuses when things go wrong with his life:

She knew damn well who she married. I would never change.

She was jealous that I was having fun and that she had to take care of the kids.

She gave more attention to the kids than she did to me.

She's fucking crazy.

I used every one of these excuses while I was going through my divorce. It took time to realize that it was me who had caused my marriage to fall apart.

The bottom line was that if I had not drank, none of those problems would have happened.

What a simple concept to understand.

T. C., I am truly sorry for what I did to you and our family. I wish things would have turned out differently. I was such a stupid mother-fucker. When you offered to quit drinking yourself to support me if I would also quit drinking, I just laughed in your face. I should have embraced that offer and taken you up on it. However, I was too selfish, and I didn't see the future far enough ahead.

A man doesn't change his behavior unless he feels he is losing something he loves. I really loved you, and my heart broke during our divorce. But, in retrospect, losing you made me realize that I needed to change my life and my behavior. You made me realize that my alcoholism was the root cause of most of the problems in my life.

Thank you, T. C. I never meant to hurt you, but I know I did. I am trying to be a good father to the kids just like you have been such a fantastic mother to them.

I have a lot of catching up to do.

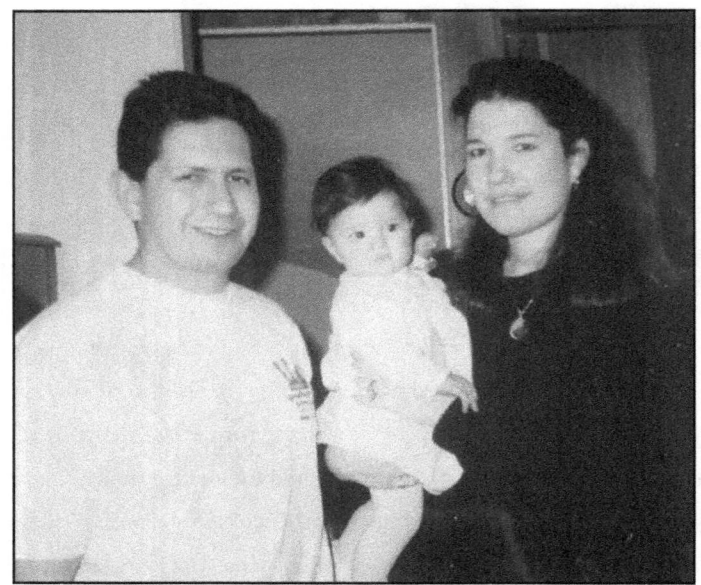

T.C., Sarah and I during a happy moment.

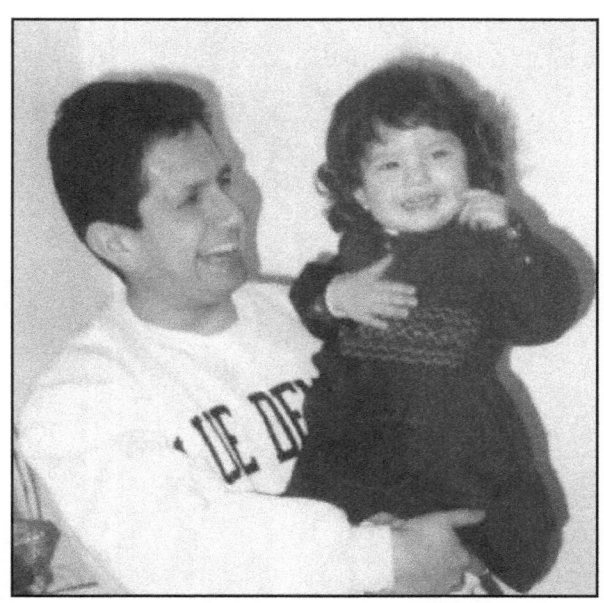

Sarah and I having a nice laugh.

HOW I STOPPED DRINKING: THE FORMULA

Approximate Date: July 2004

AFTER MY FIRST AA meeting, I was at a major crossroads in my life. The thoughts and goals I had were fairly clear in my head. I knew that I wanted to keep my marriage and my family together. And I knew that if I continued to drink, that goal would be impossible. But I also thought that not drinking would be impossible. Not drinking was never an option for me. I thought there was always another way. Time was always on my side when it came to controlling or disguising my alcoholism. However, T. C. had thrown a major monkey wrench into my usual plan of action. I had to figure out another way.

The following is the formula that worked for me and that led me to sobriety. I cannot say that this formula will work for others. But, if you are reading this, it might give you a head start in the right direction you need to take in order to work on your drinking problem.

GET MAD

Do you want to stop?

First and foremost: you have to *want* to stop drinking. It seems like a very simple concept, but it is extremely complex.

If you are stopping for a woman, it is not going to work.

If you are stopping for a man, it is not going to work.

If you are stopping for your kids, it is not going to work.

If you are stopping because of your career, it is not going to work.

If you are stopping because your family has had it with you, it is not going to work.

If you are stopping because the legal system tells you to stop, it is not going to work.

Insert any other reason in the world—it is not going to work.

The only way this will work is if **you** make a decision to want to stop **for you**.

YOU want to end this shit that is fucking up your life.

YOU don't want to wake up with a hammerhead headache in the morning.

YOU don't want to continue to fuck up your relationship with your kids.

YOU don't want to continue to be a fuck-up at your job.

YOU don't want to waste the entire day away being hung over.

YOU don't want to say something stupid at a party that embarrasses your wife.

YOU don't want to get a DUI.

YOU don't want to go to jail.

YOU don't want to wake up in a hospital strapped to a bed.

YOU want others to be proud of you.

YOU want to make the commitment to improve.

Get **MAD** (MAKE A DECISION—get the acronym?).

Once you have made the decision, the rest is easy—very easy. However, that decision is the hardest decision that you will ever have to make in your life. That decision will turn your life around. That decision will fuck with your head and your mind. That decision will make you love yourself and make you hate yourself. That decision will save your life— trust me on this one. I am no doctor, but I am an expert in this field.

My decision was made the second I announced that I was an alcoholic at my first AA meeting. I never believed it until I spoke those words out loud to a group of people. The monkey was finally off my back. My secret was no longer a secret. That was so hard for me to admit. The reason it was hard was because I knew the fun was going to be over.

I realized that all of the fun and all of the recognition that I had received from drinking was finally going to come to an end. I had to figure out a way to live without my best friend and my crutch. I had to figure out a way to live without my trusty alcohol.

WHAT THE FUCK WAS I GOING TO DO NOW?

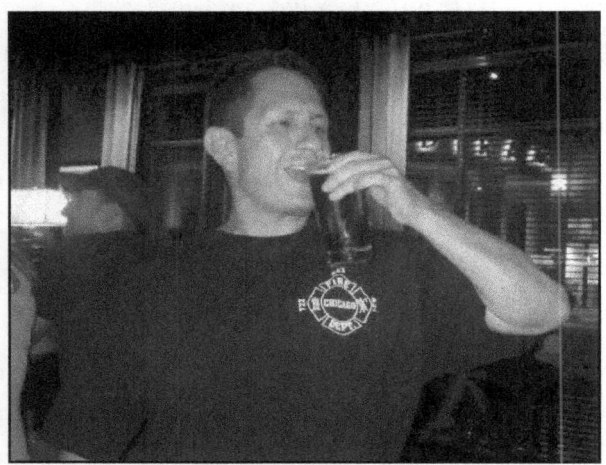

It's about to go down!

WHAT DOES IT MEAN
TO GET MAD?

HOW MANY TIMES have you woken up in the morning and said to yourself, "Why the fuck did I do that?" "Why the fuck did I say that?" I can absolutely guarantee with 100 percent certainty that every morning you wake up where you did not drink the night before, you will never say to yourself, "I wish I would have gotten fucked up last night." The moment you wake is the apex of your daily sobriety. (Apex means the "height" or the "top" of your daily sobriety for those of you reading this in prison.) You actually feel great about yourself. You know that nothing happened the night before that caused grief or harm in your life. Hey, the problems in life are all still there, but they sure as fuck did not get any worse. Let me repeat that:

THE PROBLEMS DO NOT
GET ANY FUCKING WORSE.

You know what you are up against, and you do not have that horrific hangover to make those problems seem even worse. You can now actually tackle your problems with a clear mind. Sobriety does not eliminate your problems; sobriety makes it easier for you to solve them.

I have attempted to get sober over a hundred times in my life. I have tried everything, including:

DRINKING on weekends only.

DRINKING on special occasions only.

DRINKING dark alcohol only.

DRINKING beer only.

DRINKING shots only.

DRINKING after 6 p.m. only.

DRINKING with the ninety-degree rule, which means that when you drink a bottle of beer, you cannot have the bottle go over ninety degrees in relation to your mouth. My ex-wife T. C. had me on that rule for a while. It didn't work.

DRINKING vodka and gin only.

NO SHOTS.

DRINKING when I eat only.

Never **DRINKING** at home.

Never **DRINKING** before noon.

Never **DRINKING** scotch.

Only **DRINKING** scotch.

This is going to be one of the hardest things to understand about my book and my formula. This was the most difficult concept for me to grasp about sobriety. This is a tough concept but 100 percent necessary:

YOU CAN NEVER DRINK AGAIN FOR THE REST OF YOUR LIFE.

Do you understand this concept? Never means never. If you cannot handle this, then just put this fucking book down and throw it away. This book is not for you. If you would like to save your life and you are heading down the same path that I was, then please continue to keep reading because it will be worth it.

We have all heard of the concept "one day at a time," right? On a daily basis, this is a great way to tackle your sobriety. Some people even have to take "one hour at a time" or even "one minute at a time." Sobriety is such a delicate and difficult concept to achieve. However, you must understand that sobriety means that you can never drink for the rest of your life. You must put your arms around this concept, or it will simply just not work. Your life consists of seconds, minutes, hours, days, weeks, months, and years. You only have one lifetime. You can choose to drink, or you can choose not to drink.

When you get **MAD**, you have chosen "one lifetime at a time."

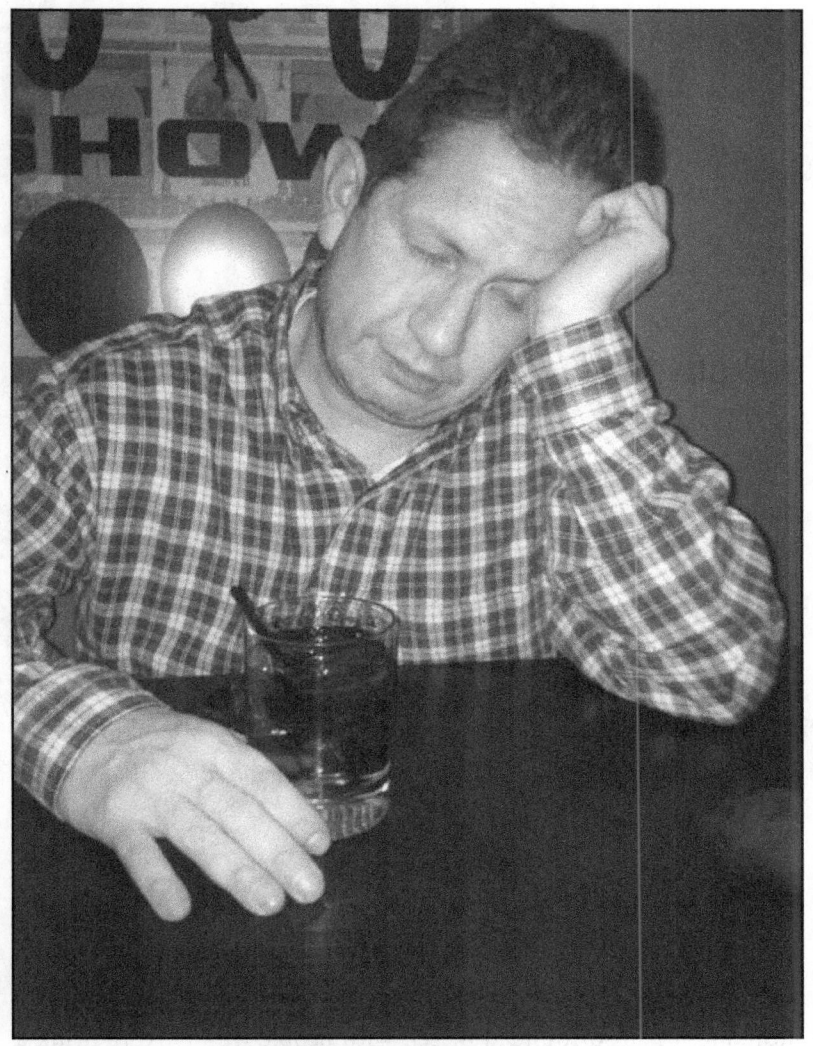

Holy shit. Do I have problems.

NOBODY GIVES A SHIT

Approximate Date: Forever

I NEVER IMAGINED a life without drinking. I believed drinking defined me. I thought drinking made me funny. I thought drinking made people want to be friends with me. I thought the amount of my drinking had a direct correlation with how much people liked me. All of my beliefs were huge fallacies. The exact opposite is true. The people who truly care about you are the ones whom you hurt time and time again with your drinking—and they are usually your family. The people who approach you and want to talk to you about your drinking problem are the smartest and most caring people in your life. You should listen to them. These are the people who speak up about the things that you are too blind to see.

When you are drinking, you surround yourself with people who really do not care what you do with your life; they only care about making themselves feel better through you. Alcoholics do not want to be bothered by people who tell them that they have a problem. My entire life, I had surrounded myself with people who liked to drink a lot. And now I had to change my thinking and behavior.

Let's face the facts, not a lot of good stories start with: "So I was enjoying a glass of water at the library the other day . . . " Now that I was trying to remain sober, I had to learn to create a life that had to be entertaining for myself without drinking. At first, I thought this was an impossible task.

How the fuck can I have fun at a Cubs game without drinking?
How the fuck can I have fun at a bar without doing shots?
How the fuck can I go to a party without guzzling a bottle of scotch?
How is anyone going to fucking like me?
It took a little while, but I got all the answers I needed.

Assume you are at a Cubs game with four of your buddies, and it is your turn to buy a round of drinks. You go down to the concession stand, and you get four Miller Lites and one bottled water. Yes, the whole process is going to be very expensive, but at least you are having that water. You are controlling your own destiny. If you're worried about what your friends will think of you when they find out you are drinking water, I have a little secret to share with you:

NOBODY GIVES A SHIT!

Enjoy your water and shut your mouth. You will be able to drive home and not worry about getting pulled over by the police.

Let's say you are at a bar and your friends are lining up shots of tequila and they pour one for you. I have a great response for your friends:

"No thank you. Ice water, please."

It takes more of a man to say no to that one shot than it takes to drink ten shots in a row. That concept took a long time for me to understand, but it is so true. Worry about yourself. You are the only one who can control your life.

NOBODY GIVES A SHIT!

Imagine yourself at a party, and everyone is drinking. That scenario was a complete nightmare for me. What was I going to do? How was I going to talk? Were people going to ignore me? Were people going to think that I was weird because I was not drinking?

Answer: have a glass of water or a soda. The conversation you are having with another person is exactly the same. Being drunk does not improve the quality of the conversation, and you will be able to drive home safely. And the girls do not get better looking as the night progresses.

NOBODY GIVES A SHIT!

Every year, on July 15, I organize a sobriety dinner to celebrate myself. I announce it on Facebook. I send a text to everyone whom I want to attend the dinner at least ten days in advance. I also send follow-up texts to those same people about three days before the dinner, and then a final text the night before the dinner. These dinners are a big deal to me, and I make sure everyone is aware that they are a big deal.

Do you know how many people would acknowledge my sobriety anniversary if I do not mention it to them first or if they do not see it on social media? The answer is zero—and that probably includes my own children. And it does not make them bad people. It just means that people worry about their own lives. People need to be constantly reminded that your sobriety is important to you. You have to create your own buzz about your sobriety because no one else will do it for you. Sobriety is truly important to only one person—you.

NOBODY ELSE GIVES A SHIT.

The bars and the parties and the concerts and the large gatherings are actually the easiest times to remain sober for me. They are constant reminders that this is not what I want in my life. And the longer I remain sober, the more affirmation I receive that the drinking life is not for me anymore. It is only when I am alone that the drinking thoughts start to creep into my head. Being alone is not easy. Make sure you have a solid support of family and friends behind you to keep you on your sober course. They are the ones who will get you through your tough times when you ask for their help.

THEY ACTUALLY MIGHT GIVE A SHIT.

ARE THESE DRINKNG STORIES BULLSHIT?

Approximate Date: July 1979 to present

THERE HAVE BEEN many people who have questioned the legitimacy of my drinking stories throughout the years. I have one question for all of the detractors—who fucking cares? I have learned throughout this process that every single drinking story I've heard from my sixteen years of AA meetings, from my life experiences, and mostly from all of my friends, are exactly the same—and I mean exactly the same. The only difference is what you do about it.

Everyone drinks to excess at one point in their lives. Everyone has had embarrassing moments; everyone has done things they have regretted tremendously while drunk. You cannot take it back. I think the difference is that at some point, something goes off in your head that says, "Enough."

FUCK this.
FUCK waking up with a hammerhead headache.
FUCK being too scared to answer the phone.
FUCK being an embarrassment to your kids.

FUCK being an embarrassment to yourself.

FUCK not remembering a thing from the night before.

FUCK screwing up a relationship that meant the world to you.

FUCK screwing up an opportunity to get a really good job.

FUCK spending a shitload of money on nothing.

FUCK constantly thinking of stopping this lifestyle.

FUCK hiding your breath in the morning from people.

FUCK missing work due to booze.

FUCK not being able to be who you can be due to something
that controls you.

FUCK this.

Now my life is better.

ANYBODY WANT TO QUESTION THIS?

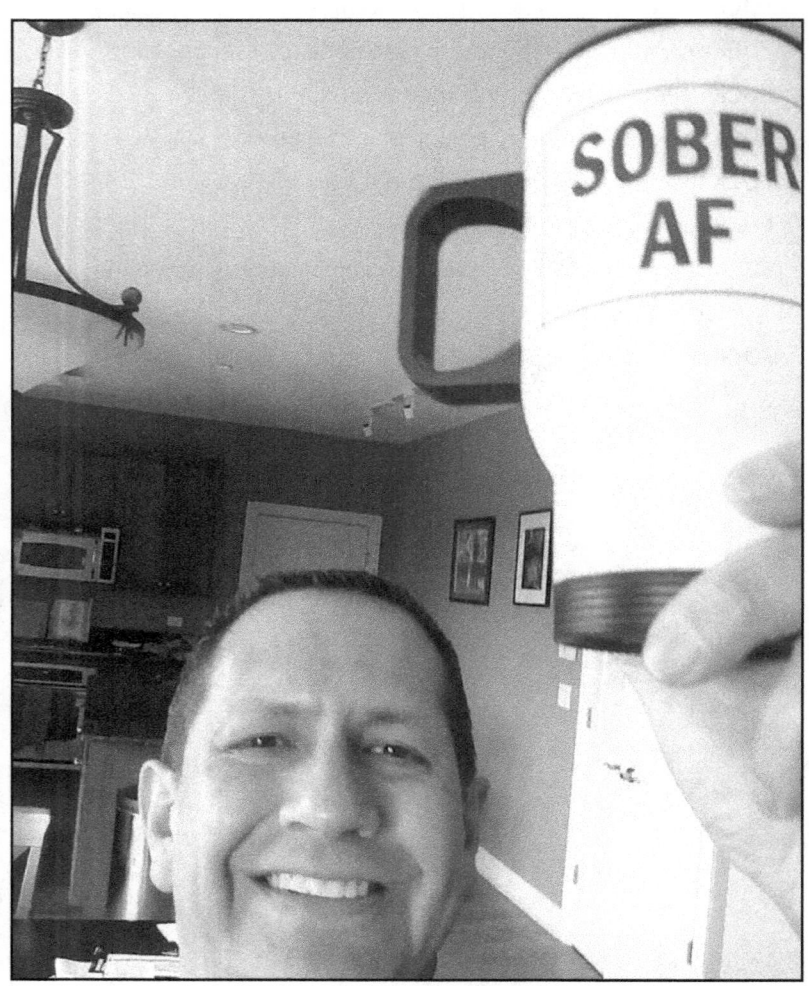

Sober As Fuck

TEMPTATION

Approximate Date: Daily

ALCOHOL IS CUNNING, baffling, and powerful. That is a major phrase in the world of Alcoholics Anonymous. What the fuck does it mean?

I currently have a shitload of alcohol in my condo. The picture of the bottles below was taken at six o'clock the morning of this writing (January 7, 2019). It's like I fuck with myself. Do I have the power to stop? Can I resist this shit? Will things ever get so bad that I will turn to this again?

When I got sober in 2004, I was going through the toughest time of my life (divorce). That was when I needed alcohol the most. But were things that bad even when I drank? I had a great job, and I lived in a great house. I had three wonderful kids. They are now twenty, twenty-four, and twenty-six years old. They are adults. Drinking is a part of their lives now; they will not really care if I drink. They have their own lives to live. I initially got sober to get my wife back, but she is not coming back. She is happy and has her own life to live. So, who the fuck cares? Who the fuck am I hurting now with my actions?

In the grand scheme of things, I think a couple of drinks are not going to kill me. I am not really an alcoholic if I have alcohol in my house, right? I learned that a "real" alcoholic hides alcohol in his house. I have never done that.

I am open and notorious with my stash. My bottles are ready to go if I need them. Nobody would ever find out. I just shouldn't drive; that would not be a good idea. The drinking and driving was what exposed me sixteen years ago when I fucking crashed my car. If I had not driven that night, fuck, I would still be married today and I would still be happy—right?

WRONG.

Everything is wrong with those paragraphs. My sobriety is everything to me. I used to have a calendar in which I would mark a red X for every day of my sobriety. My sobriety is why I am writing this paragraph at six o'clock in the morning when I should be working and trying to make money. My sobriety is why I'm trying to help at least one person with their drinking problem who might have similar crazy thoughts like these.

And, let's say I do start drinking at home, and I need more. I would hop in my car and get more booze. Maybe I would get into an accident and kill myself, or worse, kill someone else. So, a couple of drinks *would* kill me.

Those magical words: cunning, baffling, and powerful. I learned those terms in my very first AA meeting. Now I know what the fuck those words mean.

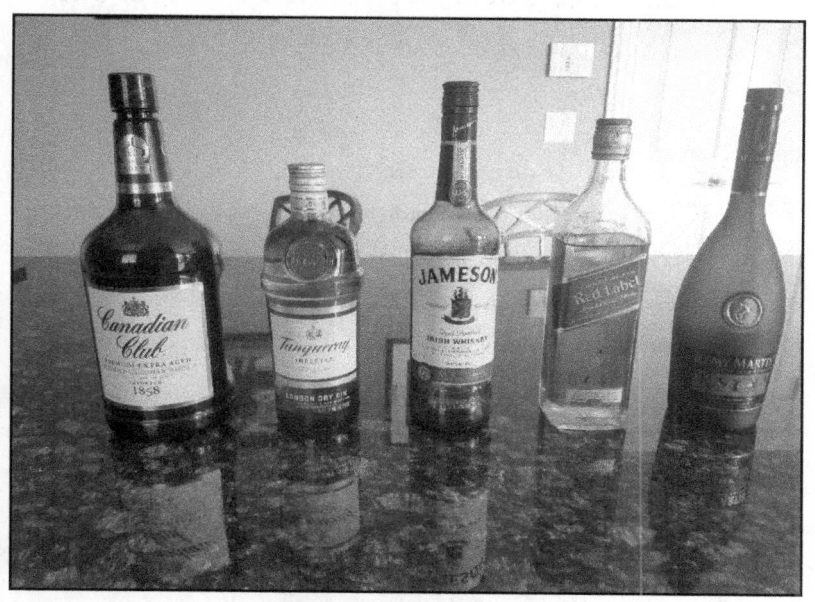

The "stash" at my condo—open and notorious—that I have never touched.

DRINKING CALENDAR

Approximate Date: July 15, 2004 to present

THE CALENDAR IS my dirty little secret.

This might sound like the stupidest idea in the world, but for me, this has a 100 percent success rate. Get a piece of paper and a pencil or a pen, and create a calendar. It doesn't matter if the calendar is a one-hour calendar or a one-year calendar.

Every day or every hour or every minute that you do not drink, mark it off with a red X. It must be a red X. I have gone to the local Walgreens at 11 p.m. looking for a red pen after I misplaced mine one night. Every day that passes is a fucking accomplishment. Be proud of that day—mark it with a red X.

Little accomplishments lead to bigger accomplishments. One day leads to one week, one week leads to one month, one month leads to six months, six months leads to one year, and one year leads to sixteen years and writing a fucking book about alcoholism.

YOU CAN DO IT.

I was helping a good friend of mine with her drinking problem, and I told her how important the calendar was for my sobriety. She created her own calendar and even texted me a picture of it. I was very impressed. It was much more neatly done than mine. It had a creative flourish to it. I was jealous of it, actually.

We would talk every day about how proud she was to mark that red X on her calendar to show off another day of her sobriety. She would even stay up till midnight just so she could mark off that day with her red X. She was quickly learning that the calendar was very important to her sobriety. I was amazed by how quickly she had embraced sobriety. She claimed her life was so much better and that she couldn't believe why she had not quit earlier in her life.

Our daily talks became only weekly talks. Then the talks became only text messages, but I still wanted to keep in touch with her to follow her through her journey. I texted her on a Sunday morning and asked how many days she had (sober days). She responded with:

"Oh, I don't even count the days anymore. I'm fine."

Wow, the red Xs had been replaced with major red flags! People have patterns. There are good patterns, and there are bad patterns. The calendar is a good pattern. When someone stops a good pattern, it is not good news. Instantly, I knew there was a problem. When you are getting sober, you know exactly how many sober days you have marked off every day—especially in your first year. When you do not use the calendar, you no longer have a visual accountability for your sobriety. You no longer have that positive feeling of marking off that red X.

My friend relapsed shortly after our last text exchange. She did not think the calendar was important to her. Maybe she relapsed and then stopped marking the calendar. Maybe she just stopped marking the calendar and then relapsed. The order does not matter. She stopped using the calendar. She stopped being accountable to herself.

Most people relapse. Most people struggle with sobriety. Most people find it extremely difficult to stop drinking. If you find yourself in a relapse situation, then you **START A NEW CALENDAR**.

The calendar is so critically important. It makes you accountable to yourself. You live to mark off that day with a red X. You will be amazed by how much you will look forward to marking that day off. Some days will be a breeze and other days will be excruciatingly difficult. I cannot emphasize how important the calendar was and is to my sobriety. If there is one "dirty little secret" to my sobriety, the calendar would be it.

The repetition of marking off the calendar is so critically important to me. Repetition became a drug and an addiction to me, just like the alcohol. I had to mark off that red X at the same time every day. The repetition became a habit. The habit then just became a part of my life. And then that habit becomes impossible to break. The same theory that created your alcoholism is used in order to create your sobriety. Just the thought of breaking my streak makes me sick to my stomach. Your worst sober day is way better than your best hung-over day.

THE CALENDAR IS IMPORTANT!

JULY 2019

Eddie DID NOT DRINK!

JULY	1 X	11	23
	2 X	12	24
	3 X	13	25
	4 X	14	26
	5 X	15	27
	6	16	28
	7	17	29
	8	18	30
	9	19	31
	10	20	
		21	
		22	

The calendar—my dirty little sobriety secret.

YOUR SOBRIETY IS A HUGE DEAL: SHOW IT OFF

Approximate Date: Forever

THIS IS THE main part of my sobriety "formula" where I veer off from the traditional Alcoholics Anonymous way of dealing with recovery.

When I was drinking, I did it pretty well. I made a conscious effort to show everyone that I wanted to drink them under the table. I wanted to show people that I was fun. I wanted to attract the attention of girls, and for that matter, guys. I wanted people to know that I was the top drinker that they would ever come across. If you went out with me for a night of drinking, you would never forget it. You would tell your friends what a great guy I was and all the crazy shit that I did while we were out.

Oh yeah, I was extremely proud of my drinking. I loved hearing the stories the next day of what I had done, as long as it wasn't too embarrassing. There wasn't a stunt that was too outrageous. I loved every minute of my drinking exploits. The only problem was those fucking consequences of my drinking.

I DID NOT enjoy getting divorced.

I DID NOT enjoy going to hospitals.

I DID NOT enjoy going to jail.

I DID NOT enjoy being the laughingstock of my community.

I DID NOT enjoy the whispers I overheard upon entering the Park Ridge Country Club.

I DID NOT enjoy crashing my car on multiple occasions.

I DID NOT enjoy disappointing my parents and my sister.

I DEFINITELY DID NOT enjoy disappointing my wife.

I DID NOT enjoy disappointing my children who had to live with me day in and day out.

So, ultimately, there comes a point in life when you must decide which way you want to go. If I continue on this path, it will surely lead to a bad situation—probably death. I really did not feel like dying. Does anyone?

My recovery began with the AA meetings. I started to be pretty vocal during my early meetings at the Main Center on Busse Highway in Park Ridge, Illinois. I was a pretty good speaker, and I loved to tell my drinking stories. People thought they were very funny. I also asked a lot of questions during other people's "talking time," which you are really not supposed to do in AA, but the head of the meeting allowed me to do it anyway.

I tried to make everyone else feel accepted. I tried to communicate: "Hey, it is okay. Do not be embarrassed whatsoever. There is not a story that is too crazy or too unbelievable. We are all alcoholics here. You are not unusual. We are all fuck-ups. And we are all here to help each other."

I started to bring burgers and pizzas to the meetings. As I stated before, I hated the fact that the only thing we had at the meetings to drink was coffee, and I hate coffee. I wanted to spice things up a little bit.

People at the meetings thought my stories were outrageous. I was actually getting positive attention from my drinking stories. I would also talk about how I felt like I was a failure to my family. I spoke of how my drinking had ruined everything that I had worked so hard to achieve. The AA meetings were a major eye-opener for me.

Jack Canfield is an author, motivational speaker, corporate trainer, and entrepreneur. He is the coauthor of the Chicken Soup for the Soul series, which has more than 250 titles and 500 million books in print in over forty languages. I have watched countless of his motivational videos. When he is about to say something important, he always says:

"Okay, write this down." (And he proceeds to give you some powerful and necessary life-changing information).

Well, here is my Jack Canfield moment.

WRITE THIS SHIT DOWN!

I came upon a major revelation: I realized the attention I thought I could only get through drinking was already available to me through sobriety. This concept was a game changer for me. I had found a way to stop drinking and still be happy and still have a purpose in my life.

Sobriety can act like a runaway train in the same way that alcoholism can. You can set up your life in the same "vicious circle," kind of way that alcohol did for you previously. Make sobriety your alcoholism. Was alcohol your obsession? It sure was for me. Now, make sobriety your new obsession.

Sobriety is such a big deal. Show it off. Getting sober has been the best possible thing I have ever done in my life, and I need to show it off! I want to maximize the number of people who know about my sobriety. I want people to know that I have worked extremely hard to get and to stay sober. I want social media to know that this is a gigantic deal. The more people who know about it, the better off you will be. Having more people know that I am sober will decrease the chances that I will ever drink again. The less people who know that I am sober, the higher the chance that I will drink again. Making a big deal about your sobriety makes you accountable to yourself.

If you do not want people to know about your sobriety, ask yourself: is it because, in the back of your mind, you are planning on drinking again and you do not want to disappoint others and yourself? Be honest with yourself.

I have tried to counsel many people on their drinking problems, and I find that a major red flag to their sobriety is when they do not want me to say anything to anyone about their struggles. There is still a stigma that alcoholism should not be spoken about and that it is a private and "family" matter. Well, I agree that the alcoholism part of the story should be private—understandably, nobody wants others to know the destruction and disappointment that their alcoholism caused. However, the sobriety part of the story is the exact opposite. Sobriety is the light at the end of the tunnel. The light should shine brightly for everyone to see, and you are the only one who can make it shine.

SOBRIETY DINNERS

July 2005 to the Present

"LET'S HAVE A party for your sobriety!"

After my car accident on July 15, 2004, I started to stack some alcohol-free days together. I had one month of sobriety. I felt pretty good. The AA meetings were helping. And I had been in so much legal and family trouble over my car accident that I wasn't getting any pressure to drink. My friends were actually scared to ask me to go out with them.

[**Note to others:** this is a strong indication that you may have a drinking problem.]

I began going to two AA meetings a week in my first year of sobriety. I loved the meetings and could not wait for the part of the meeting where we could start talking about our own experiences so I could "show off" my drinking stories. I am fully aware that this does not sound like the optimal way to get sober. The glorification of alcoholism and drinking might not work for everyone. But it worked for me. I found a reason to "look forward" to the meetings. The disease is one that messes with your head as much as it messes with your body. Sometimes you need to rewire things mentally in order to combat the disease. The important result was that I went to the meetings. I never went to a meeting that ended in a negative result.

ONE MONTH BECAME SIX MONTHS.

At the time, I was still considering going back to "casual drinking" once the heat from my family and the law came off my back. However, this sobriety thing was not as terrible as I had thought it would be. I was counting each day that I stayed sober. I marked each day with a red X on my calendar. It would be a shame to fuck up my streak.

My one year of sobriety was soon approaching. I knew the enormity of what being one year sober meant for me. This was the longest that I had ever even dreamed of staying sober. What the fuck was I going to do to mark this momentous occasion?

Two of my friends, Erica Tan and Raquel Baldwin, had this fantastic idea of having a "Sobriety Dinner" on the night of my one-year sobriety anniversary, which was July 15, 2005. We would invite people to eat and drink and speak and celebrate. We would treat it just like a normal party, except that we were celebrating my sobriety.

The first Annual Eddie Arana Sobriety Dinner was at a restaurant called Ballo on Dearborn and Illinois Street in downtown Chicago. There were about thirty people in attendance, a combination of friends and family. People drank a lot at the party. I didn't care. I actually encouraged it. This was definitely a reason to celebrate. Just because I wasn't drinking didn't mean that I wanted my friends to stay sober. I came prepared with a speech, which I read after dinner. People became really emotional during the speech, including myself.

It was a very successful night. I was extremely proud of myself. Several people had also made speeches that inspired me to keep this sobriety thing going. It was happening. I was getting that same feeling of euphoria that I used to get when I was drinking! Is this fucking possible? What the fuck? Had I unlocked the secret to life? I could still have fun without drinking?

If you are a problem drinker, I am sure this is one of your biggest fears about sobriety. Can I still enjoy myself without the booze? The answer is a definitive yes. You can do whatever you put your mind to. Alcohol is not a necessary part of your life if you do not want it to be. I remember going home the night of that party and thinking to myself, Holy fuck. I figured it out. Life can still be fun. I am getting the same kind of attention that I used to get. However, this time it is for a good reason, not for a disaster.

The problem with sobriety is that it takes a while. It is not a fly-by-night operation. You must be committed to it, or it will not work. You can only realize the important things about sobriety when you have been sober enough to realize them. It is very confusing. For example, these sobriety dinners are a lot of fun. What makes them fun? The answer is the people who attend, the occasion that they represent, and the memories that they create.

I have looked back on my life and seen how many major events I had been so drunk through that I barely remember them. The Cubs playing at Wrigley Field has nothing to do with drinking; I am there to watch a baseball game and to cheer on the Cubs. Going to someone's wedding has nothing to do with drinking; I am there to share in the union of two people who want me to be a part of their special day. A Christmas party has nothing to do with drinking; the event celebrates a holiday that comes once a year. A Fourth-of-July picnic has nothing to do with drinking; it is meant to celebrate the independence of our country. A retirement party has nothing to do with drinking; the party is designed to celebrate someone who is finally stopping work after having worked for most of their life.

The reason for each event is not based on drinking. However, I made them about drinking. I created that cause and effect. And the longer you remain sober, the more you realize that the drinking was an unnecessary part of the event. When you are a drunk, you have very little memories of huge life events or parties and celebrations because you had been so fucked up that you have forgotten about them.

The Chicago Cubs won the World Series in 2016. I watched Game 7 by myself in my living room. I celebrated that night as if the Cubs had won the World Series (oh wait, they did). My point is that if I had been drinking, the only memory I probably would have had about that night would be that the Cubs had won, but I would have had no idea about the other details of the game. That was the single biggest moment in my life as a Cubs fan, and I can honestly say that I relished every moment of that victory. I know how fucked up I would have gotten had I been drinking, and I would have been so pissed off at myself.

The following year's second Annual Eddie Arana Sobriety Dinner was located at the Park Ridge Country Club, the site of my last drink. Just like the first year, we had a nice dinner, and then came the speeches. This time, I wanted my speech to be the last of the speeches. I have always wanted to have the last word. It was also a great party. However, the bill was not great. The party cost me about $2,500. I was getting charged four dollars for bottled water! Let's just say that this was the last time my sobriety dinner would be at the Park Ridge Country Club. The staff and the atmosphere were second to none, but my bank account took a major hit.

The rest of my sobriety dinners up until the present day have been at two Peruvian restaurants in Chicago—Ay Ay Picante on North Elston Avenue and Ceviche on West Diversey Parkway. I love Peruvian food, and both restaurants are BYOB, which cuts down on the bill considerably. If you want to drink at my sobriety dinner, go right ahead. However, you will have to bring your own liquor.

The whole key to my sobriety was replacing the buzz and every other "benefit" that used to come along with my drinking. This was what I thought:

ALCOHOL made me popular.
ALCOHOL made me funny.
ALCOHOL made me able to talk to women.
ALCOHOL made me say and do things that I would never do sober.

I WAS DEAD WRONG.

The alcohol did not make me popular. I am sure that it turned a lot of people off. Who the fuck wants to see and talk to a guy who is constantly making a fool of himself?

Alcohol did not make me funny. I am just as fucking funny when I am sober! I even remember all of my jokes better. What a fallacy.

Alcohol did not make me talk to women. Alcohol just made me say stupid shit to women. I had no idea that most women do not like to be around a man who is drunk.

Again, it takes sobriety to learn and understand all of this. It is like a vicious circle, but in a good way. You drink, and you make all of these fucking mistakes. You get sober, and you learn from all of your mistakes. But it takes time. It takes years. This cannot be done in one day. It takes steps, and it takes willpower.

Do you want to improve yourself?

Do you want to stay married?

Do you want to stay at your job?

Do you want to stay healthy?

Do you want a good relationship with your friends?

Do you want a good relationship with your children?

Of course, everyone's answers are a resounding yes, correct? But that fucking alcohol has a different answer. It robs you of all of those things if you abuse it. It changes what you think is important, and it takes its own sweet time doing it. It really got me good. The key is to recognize that it has gotten you. Be honest with yourself. If you are not honest, this book will do you absolutely no good. I always had a little voice in the back of my head telling me that my drinking was not normal. I knew that I was hurting the people who really cared about me. But I didn't give a fuck.

When you start to give a fuck is when you reach out for help. I think that if you are reading this, you probably know at least one person who has a major problem with drinking. Maybe you can somehow slip this book underneath their door.

I WANT TO HELP ONE PERSON.

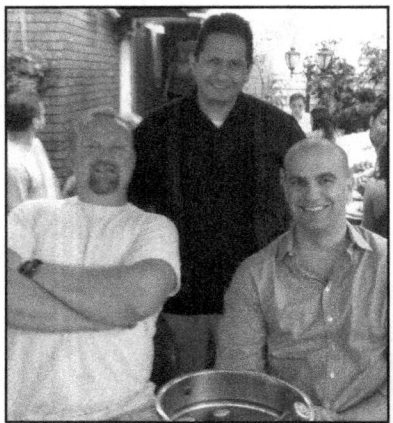

Yaki, Magoonaugh and myself.
Magoonaugh has one month more
sobriety than I do.

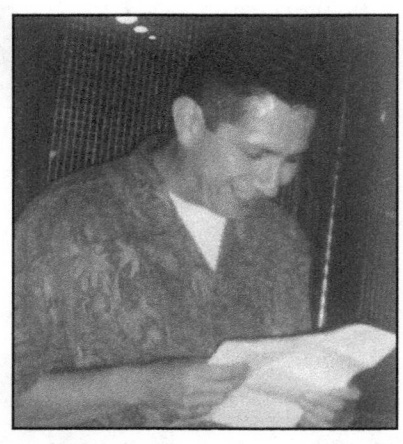

Sobriety dinner #1 taken on July 15,
2005 where I read my first speech.

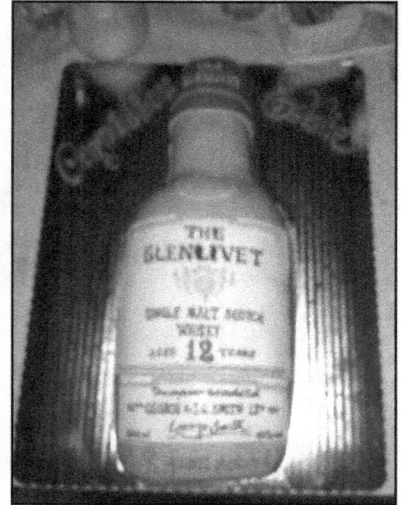

Sobriety Dinner Glen Livet Cake—
great tasting too!

TEN-YEAR SOBRIETY DINNER SPEECH

July 15, 2014

THE FOLLOWING IS a speech I gave at my ten-year sobriety dinner at my favorite Peruvian restaurant in Chicago, Ceviche. My speech is always the highlight of my dinners (I am so arrogant!).

Here it is:

Welcome to the tenth Annual Eddie Arana Sobriety Dinner. I want to thank the staff of Ceviche—Chicago's brand-new premier Peruvian restaurant serving Logan Square's finest collection of pimps, hoes, alcoholics, and heroin addicts. It is a pleasure to be here, and hopefully, this can be the site of the eleventh Annual Eddie Arana Sobriety Dinner— if there is one. I am also going to try to get through this speech without swearing, as my good friend Tina Anderson is opposed to it and says that the story can be told without swearing. We will see how that works out.

I want to thank Tim Calcagno for his tremendous skills and for agreeing to emcee tonight. T-Cal and I have become quite close the last few months or so. He does not know this, but this friendship did not just "happen" by accident. I sought him out specifically for this night.

Once he gets started, he cannot stop. Nobody else would be willing to do this emcee job. Well, let's face the facts: I do not have any friends who can even string six words together to form a sentence, much less host an event of this magnitude. Quick T-Cal story if you have a minute:

I like to walk every day in order to exercise so I can lose weight and not look like a sphere. A few Sundays ago, I asked T-Cal if he would like to walk with me. He was agreeable to the aforementioned work-out. I picked him up at his modest multimillion-dollar Park Ridge condo at 7:15 a.m. We proceeded to "walk" and I returned home at 10:15 a.m. because I had to get to breakfast with my Peruvian family. So, if you are all following correctly, that is an elapsed time of three hours. We walked a total of one-eighth of a mile, which is the equivalent of one city block. He had to come to a complete stop when telling one of his "stories" using wild hand and arm gestures to further illustrate his point. At one point, we had to sit down because he insisted that this particular part of the story needed me to be sitting because of the emotional effect it was going to have on me. We were in Starbucks for over an hour and a half talking to everybody in there. To make a long story short, I will never ask him to "work out" ever again.

I would also like to thank each and every one of you for coming to this dinner. I joke around all the time, but tonight has really meant a lot to me. I know everybody has busy schedules, and I know that people have a lot better things to do than to be here listening to this. And I hope that these two words will keep people coming back for years to come. These two words are "free food."

Most of you have heard all of my drinking stories through Facebook, which is a form of social media that weak people such as myself have become addicted to. I really do not want to go over the stories of urinating and defecating and vomiting all over myself again. I think they are rather disgusting and do not belong in a family atmosphere such as this. But the whole reason that I am here is pretty simple. Actually, every story is exactly the same, so I can summarize it quite easily:

I would make a plan to go out drinking at some point during the day. I knew full well that this plan was going to somehow negatively impact my family. I did not care. I never cared. It was not important to me. The alcohol was the most important part to me. This same story happened on thousands of days and nights with me. A very good friend of mine, who will remain anonymous, once told me that true alcoholism is not taking the first drink; it is the thought that precedes the first drink. That little concept is really the root of alcoholism—so simple to understand yet so impossible to stop.

I ended up in the hospital with a car that was totaled and a family that was tired of picking up the pieces to a life that I had shattered. I remember lying in the hospital room like it was yesterday, thinking to myself: What have I done? How had I let it get this bad? How am I going to spin this so it doesn't seem so bad? When am I going to be able to drink again? I know I have to pretend to stop drinking for a while so I can get my family to buy into my bullshit for a little bit, then I can get back to normal partying.

I liken myself to a modern-day idiot savant—emphasis on the idiot part. If any one of you have ever been out to dinner with me, you know that I might ask, "Did we order yet?" four or five times during a meal. I really do not know why I do this, and I really do not know if we have ordered yet, but I think the mere asking of the question makes me feel good for some reason. I love repetition. I like to do the same thing over and over and over again. When I drank, I liked to do the same thing also. I drank till I was so drunk that I passed out or I could not physically handle it anymore. Eventually, the consequences beat you up. To borrow another AA saying, you get sick and tired of being sick and tired.

I decided not to drink for one week after the accident. That would do it. I would be just fine in one week. Most of my wounds would have been healed, and I would have a new car by then. So, I asked T. C., "Hey, let's go grab some dinner and I will have just ONE drink to celebrate that this whole thing is behind us." T. C. said, "No, you are NOT going to have ONE more drink. You are an alcoholic. If you have one more drink, I am gone." So, I was like, fuck this isn't good. Maybe it will just have to be a little longer than one week. I gave it one month. I even started going to AA meetings and got my thirty-day coin. I actually felt like I had accomplished something, and the other drunks in AA congratulated me. I thought it was pretty cool, and I started to go to two meetings a week basically because I thought they were funny and I could mentally make fun of them.

The next milestone was a hundred days. I had put a big red X on a calendar for each day that I was sober as well. Every night at midnight, I would cross that X. Every day with that X made me feel good. It was almost like I didn't want to break the streak. I had never been a hundred days sober since I was eighteen years old, and I was forty-one years old at the time. I was still going out with the same group of friends. Thank god that I was such a horrible, nasty drunk who got into so many problems that my friends hardly ever encouraged me to drink. Next thing I knew, we were approaching the six-month mark. Now things were getting interesting. Half a year. Not a drop of alcohol. I was still pretty determined to be able to eventually drink casually and socially—because we all know how well that worked out in the past.

People were starting to take notice, and I was starting to tell people that I hadn't drank in six months. The reaction was so positive that I felt that I should not stop.

Do you know how people text acronyms like LOL (laughing out loud), SMH (shaking my head), WTF (What the fuck?), or FU (fuck you)? I had created an acronym that I would text to people all the time. It is PATM. Does anybody know what that is? Yes! Pay attention to me. I love attention. I am what is commonly known as an attention whore. When I was drinking, I got that attention. I was the life of the party. I was the guy who was going to do that crazy thing that nobody thought I could do. I was the man with the plan. Nobody could touch me when I was drinking. I went hard every time I drank, and I let everyone know about it. It was very difficult to give up that life because that was all I knew and that was all I ever wanted.

A very funny thing happened on my way to one year of sobriety. I was getting the same kind of attention. However, it was positive attention. I decided to have a big dinner for my one-year sobriety date. People brought presents and cards, and everybody was congratulating me. My kids were all there, and they seemed so proud of me. I loved that attention. I wanted more of that attention. If I drank, I would no longer have that attention. Everything would get all fucked up again if I drank. I did not want to disappoint anybody, especially my children, who had seen the worst of my alcoholism. I was starting to get happy again about life. It has been the best decision I have ever made in my life. One year is now ten years, and I hope ten years will become a lifetime.

THANK YOU VERY MUCH.

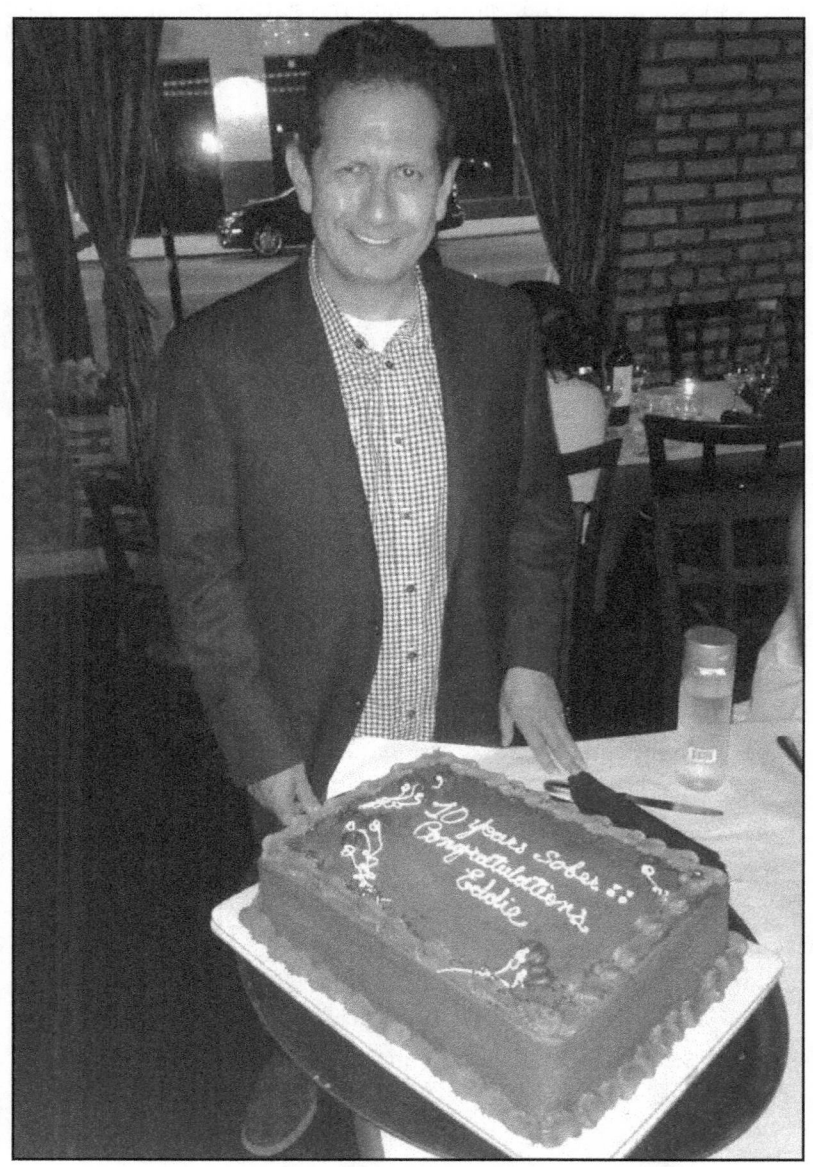

10 Year Sobriety Chocolate Cake—Well Deserved!

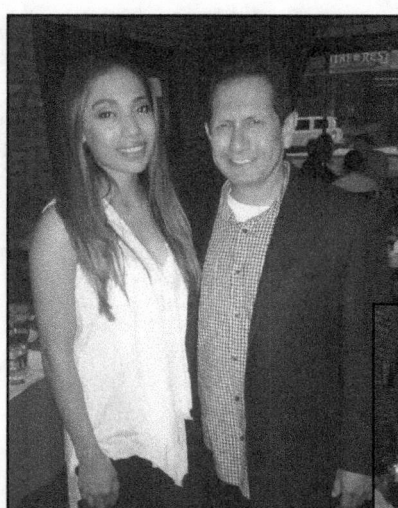

Julie Casimiro and myself celebrating sobriety!

T.C. and I and a bottle of Voss!

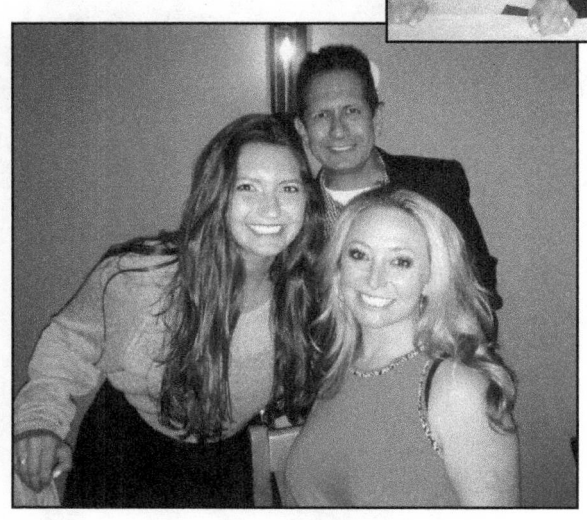

Kiki Cardelli, my daughter Sarah, and myself having fun!

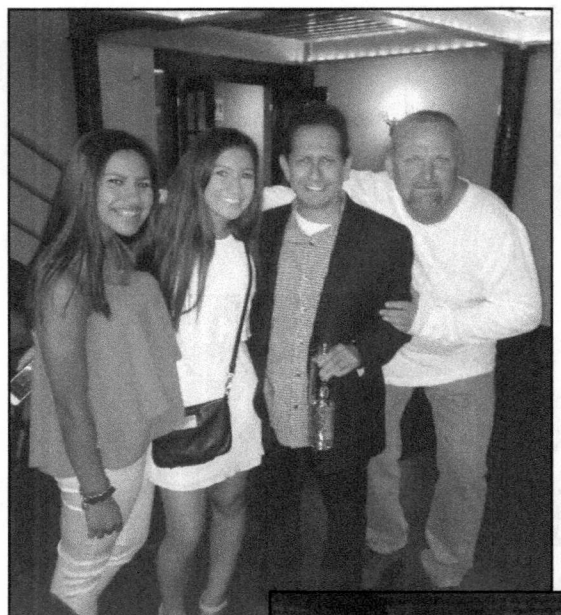

Gabby Arroyo, my daughter Isabelle, myself, and Yaki at Ceviche

Mike Milazzo, myself, and the late, great Timmy Markowski celebrating not drinking.

KARA CARDELLI

October 2004 to the Present

"C'MON, YOU'RE MEXICAN. Make me a fucking quesadilla!"

One of my gigantic fears about sobriety was that I would never be able to talk to women for the rest of my life. How the fuck was I ever going to be in a relationship again without my trusty alcohol? The booze made me funny, and the booze made me likeable. Without my alcohol, I would crawl into a corner and sit in a fetal position for the rest of my life. What the fuck was I going to do? The beginning of my sobriety coincided with the end of my marriage. This was a true disastrous situation for me. I was in a complete depression about my divorce, and on top of that, I had this sobriety that I had to work so hard to maintain.

I had organized a dinner for some friends at one of my favorite restaurants in Chicago called Ay Ay Picante. They served delicious and mouth-watering Peruvian food. My very good friend and mentor of sorts, Max Waisvisz, attended the dinner with his girlfriend, and future wife, Carla Rodriguez. He was the owner of Gold Coast Tickets in Chicago, which was the city's most successful ticket broker company.

I had just started my own ticket broker business, and Max had been an invaluable asset for advice and guidance. I was seated next to Carla, and we started to talk. I told her how I had just gotten divorced and that I loved to drink single malt scotch. I guess I failed to mention to Carla that I was also about sixteen months sober at the time. She immediately got on the phone with her roommate, Kara Cardelli, who was vacationing and partying in Miami at the time. "Hey, Kara, I am sitting at dinner with a guy whom you are going to like. He loves to drink scotch, and he is also a ticket broker!"

Kara and I made plans to go out with a group of my friends for the first time on the Wednesday night before Thanksgiving, which is typically the busiest bar night of the year in Chicago.

BRILLIANT MOVE, EDDIE.

When I first met Kara, I was floored. She was young and drop-dead gorgeous with a fantastic sense of humor. I was fucked, and not in the good way. How was I going to be able to hold a conversation with this rock star? I could only talk to girls when I was drunk or on my way to getting drunk. What the fuck was I going to do? It took Kara about two rounds of drinks to figure out that I was not drinking.

Kara asked, "Wait a second, Carla told me that you loved to drink scotch! Why the fuck aren't you drinking?"

I told her that I was sixteen months sober and that I didn't really plan on drinking for a while. I also told her that drinking had fucked up my life and that my sobriety was extremely important to me. I was shocked at Kara's reaction. She didn't seem to give a shit. She seemed pleased that she could have a designated driver for the night.

We went to five or six different bars that night. Kara liked to drink Dewar's Scotch whisky. I was so jealous of her being able to drink. Kara reminded me of what I loved about drinking. She really enjoyed it. She made a big deal about it. She was popular. She was the life of the party. I remember that night like it was yesterday.

Kara and I spent the next six months together after that night. We were inseparable. We would see each other almost every day and night. She was actually proud of the fact that I did not drink. She never made a big deal about my sobriety. I was in shock that someone in this world actually wanted to spend time with me as a sober person. She made me feel like if I did drink, it would be a major disappointment to her. I liked not having the pressure to drink. It was like having a major weight off of my shoulder.

THERE WAS HOPE FOR LOSERS LIKE ME!

My sobriety did not stop Kara from drinking whatsoever. This actually made me feel very good. I would have felt a great deal of guilt if I had been with someone who felt that they couldn't drink in front of me. I was the one with the drinking problem, not Kara. This was such an important time during my recovery. I felt that I could still find happiness without drinking. What a major breakthrough!

The first week that we started hanging out together, I was driving Kara back to her apartment. It was about 4:30 a.m., and Kara asked if I wanted to come in for a bit. I explained to her that I had to be up at 5:45 a.m., which was in about an hour an fifteen minutes. I liked to get up early to work. My schedule was very important to me. But she didn't give a shit about what time I had to be up, so I agreed to come in to her apartment.

Once we were inside, Kara announced, "I'm starving! Can you make me a quesadilla?" I told her that I really did not know how to cook and that I didn't know how to make a quesadilla. She shot back, "C'mon, you're Mexican. Make me a fucking quesadilla!" I explained to her, "Actually, Kara, I am not Mexican. I am Peruvian." She replied, "Same shit! Make me a quesadilla!"

I was so mad at that comment that I immediately left. I don't think I even said goodbye. How dare she say that to me. Kara tried to call me for the next couple of days, and I either did not answer or I was very short with her. She finally asked me what was wrong, and I told her about our conversation about the quesadilla. She started laughing hysterically. She apologized and explained that she had been drunk that night and hadn't meant it.

I began to think to myself how many stupid fucking things I had said and done when I was drunk. Then I thought about her comment, which I suddenly found hilarious. "Same shit" was funny! Thinking that Mexicans and Peruvians were the same was funny! I had lost sight of my sense of humor. You begin to see things in a different light. Sobriety teaches patience with others who drink. Sobriety teaches you not to take life so seriously. I learned to appreciate Kara's sense of humor and to not run away from it or judge it.

New Year's Eve 2005 was one that I would never forget. Kara and I went to Miami's South Beach with Max and Carla. I was dreading this weekend getaway. I had not been out of town since I had attempted sobriety, which was about twenty months ago. I hate the heat and I hate the sun and I hate water and I hate vacations. Kara enjoyed all of that kind of stuff. She enjoyed living life to the fullest. She was not afraid of anything, and she was never scared of a good time.

The weekend started off innocently enough with us just chilling in the hotel pool. Everyone was drinking and tanning and laughing, and I was a nervous wreck. This was not fun for me. When could we go back to Chicago so I could watch TV and work on making money?

When could we go to a restaurant and eat a steak and dessert? Why were people in the water? How could anyone be having fun in this environment? Oh, Kara, you need another shot of tequila? Let me go grab it for you. Do you need anything else while I am at the bar? Oh, another Dewar's on the rocks? Sounds great, I will get right on that. Where is the fucking business center so I can get on the fucking computer so I can check on my business?

Later that evening, we all went to a Snoop Dogg concert. Kara and Carla loved Snoop. This was one of my first major sobriety tests, and I was not handling it well. I felt like I was an extra in a Cheech & Chong movie. Everyone around me was either smoking weed or drinking, or both. I was in a complete state of panic. When was this fucking night going to end? Was this what sober life was like? How the fuck was I going to survive this?

SOMEONE, GET ME A GLENLIVET NEAT!

After the concert, Kara had the great idea of sneaking into a hotel swimming pool at about three o'clock in the morning. An added bonus was that we didn't have any swimming gear, so we had to go in naked. I was fucking terrified. What if someone saw us? I was naked in a fucking pool, and I was sober as fuck, and I wanted to go home! And I was with a lunatic (granted, a beautiful lunatic) who didn't want the night to end and thought it was okay to be drinking champagne in a pool at 3 a.m. Sure enough, after about forty-five minutes of being in the pool, a big, beefy security guard shone his flashlight on us and politely asked us what the fuck we were doing there.

I was flabbergasted. My worst nightmare had come true. We had been caught. But Kara thought it was the funniest thing ever. She laughed and laughed at the situation while I was mortified. I apologized to the security guard and took my naked ass out of the pool and begged Kara to do the same. After a short walk on the beach with the bottle of champagne, the night was finally over.

It took a few days for it to sink in that I needed to loosen up and enjoy life. Alcohol did not control me. I could enjoy life without it. I did not die that night. I went out of my comfort zone, and I made it through alive. I did not drink that night. It was extremely difficult, but I kept my sobriety. I was at a fucking Snoop Dogg concert, and I was skinny-dipping in a fucking hotel pool, for god's sake.

I WAS GOING TO MAKE IT!

Thank you, Kara Cardelli, for teaching me that I can still have fun and have a sense of humor without drinking. Thank you for being yourself and for showing me a great time. And thank you for convincing me that I can still talk to women without drinking.

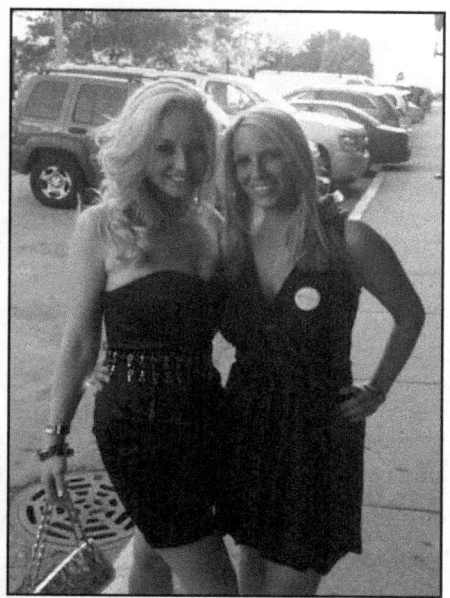

Kara Cardelli (on the left) and her friend "Whispers."

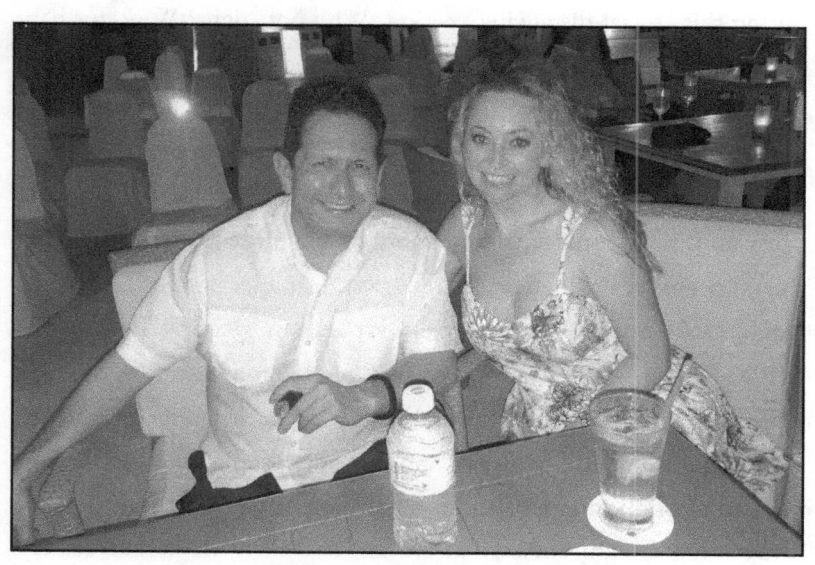

Kara and I in Cabo San Lucas, Mexico, on a vacation.

JOHN MORAN

March 17, 2020

MAJOR PROBLEM:

I am seriously considering drinking during this coronavirus pandemic. My licensed ticket broker business is in the tank. No one is buying or selling tickets during this time. I am in debt over $250,000. There is no financial relief in sight. I am stuck in my condo with nothing to do during this "social distancing" period. Why not, right? Why not have that drink or those drinks in order to feel better. A beer or a scotch would make me feel so much better right now. I know who I can call to immediately have a drink with me. I need it more than ever right now.

I am going nuts being quarantined in this fucking house by myself. I just want to get drunk just one more time in order to feel better, and then, I promise, I will go back to sobriety. Just a six pack of Miller Lite would make my problems go away for at least a couple of hours. A bottle of Glenlivet single malt scotch would last me for at least a couple of days. No one would ever know. My kids are vacationing in Cabo San Lucas right now until Saturday, and it is only Wednesday. Yes, I know I am an alcoholic and I should not be thinking like this, but these are extenuating circumstances that we are dealing with in our society. Nothing like this has ever happened before.

It is not the end of the world if I have a few drinks. No one would ever know. I don't give a fuck about my fifteen years of sobriety right now. Someone please fucking help me. Someone please tell me what to do. I am drowning! I am in a complete depression. I do not know what I am going to do with this mounting debt. I am so fucking stressed out. There are tears running down my cheek right now just writing this shit down. God, help me remain strong. I don't know what to do. Nobody is paying attention to me. I do not have a wife or a girlfriend to tell me that everything is going to be okay. My mom passed away less than two months ago. She hated my drinking. I love you so much, Mom. Where are you? I need you more than ever right now! Help me not think like this!

SOLUTION:

Fortunately for me, this is not an unusual situation, and it should not be an unusual situation for alcoholics. We have all encountered that feeling of helplessness. We sense that despair that completely takes over our mind and body. It is an uncontrollable desire to drink. Your mind begins to play tricks on you. Nothing matters except for the liquor. You can rationalize yourself into thinking that having a drink is okay and that you will be fine if you have that drink. You make yourself think that it is okay to throw all of your hard work right out the window and relapse. It is not a fun time to be sober, and you do not believe there is any way out except to have that drink.

Does this sound familiar? Thankfully, if you know what to do in these moments and who to reach out to, the feeling and the situation can be fixed—and it can be fixed relatively quickly and easily.

That day, I reached out to my friend John Moran who is an alderman in Park Ridge in addition to being a co-owner of the Moran-Havansek

Financial Group (shameless plug). I made up some bullshit that I needed to go to his office to use his scanner in order to email some documents. I also messaged him that I was not in a good place and that I wanted to drink .

John knows my history with alcoholism and understands what a problem it would be if I had a drink. I know what type of friend he is. I knew what he was going to tell me—that I was fucking crazy if I decided to have that drink. I knew that he would try everything in his power to prevent me from drinking. If you are an alcoholic, I hope and pray you have a friend like John Moran. I walked into his office and approached his desk and saw his smiling face—and everything was already better in my head. We laughed about the stock market and about our diets and bantered on with self-deprecating humor for about thirty minutes. I told him that I was going to McDonald's and asked him if he wanted a Big Mac. He looked at me like I was fucking crazy, and I left his office. That is how easily and quickly your crazy desire to drink can go away.

I got in my car and noticed that he had responded to my earlier message with exactly what I thought he would say. This was his message back to me:

"Go back. Get all of the booze in your house and bring it here. I'll hold on to it. Do you really think drinking will help you with your situation? You know that any chance you have of improving your situation goes out the fucking window when you start with that shit." I reread his text several times and I have come to the conclusion that:

A. This was a bizarre way of improving his personal alcohol stash

or

B. He was being a genuine friend and wanted to help me out.

Drunks like me need the John Morans of this world in our lives. We rely on family and friends to keep us sober. We know what they are going to say and what they are going to do. We just have to be smart enough to reach out to them when we need to hear how fucking stupid we are and before we do something really fucking stupid. The solution is not difficult at all. The difficult part is asking for the help. People actually enjoy helping others in need. Do not be afraid to ask. My family was out of town, and I needed a friend to help me that day.

I am still sober. John Moran helped me.

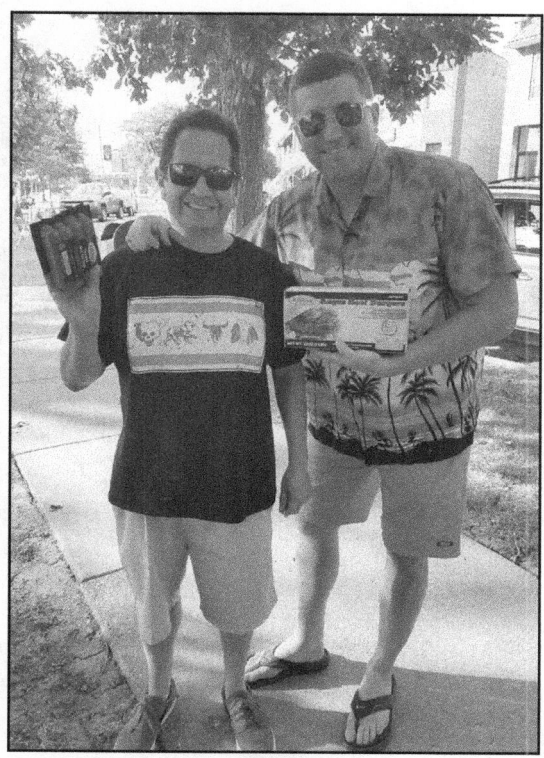

John Moran and myself goofing off in Park Ridge

ISABELLE ARANA: THE PRODIGY

January 2016 to the Present

SHE DRINKS LIKE I used to drink. This is my fault.

As an alcoholic with children, one of your big fears in life is passing the drinking "gene" on to one of your kids. My youngest daughter, Isabelle, has been an athletic and academic superstar her entire life. She has gotten straight As since fifth grade, throughout high school, and through her first three years of college. Isabelle is also a drinker. And when I say a drinker, I mean a drinker.

She started out drinking at parties and in people's basements and at music festivals and at "sleepovers" at her friends' houses. It became a running joke how much "little" Isabelle could drink. Isabelle is a small person, so a little alcohol can do a lot of damage to her small frame.

Isabelle is what is known as a blackout drunk. When she drinks, she blacks out and has very little to zero memory of what she did or what had happened to her the night or day before. This is the most dangerous type of drinking for young adults in my opinion.

Isabelle is also very funny when she drinks. She is quick with the wit and insults. People like to be around her. She reminds me of her funny and quick-witted father.

The first time you see one of your children drunk or high is surreal. You think you can be that "cool" parent who can remember what it was like when you were fifteen years old. But the pain is there. The pain of knowing that what they are doing to their bodies is not good.

It is your responsibility to make sure that she is okay. It is your responsibility to make sure she is safe from the evils of the world. It is your responsibility to make sure she remains alive long enough so you can be proud of her. There is also the guilt that you gave her the alcoholic gene. You created this part of her that will inevitably fuck up her entire life. This guilt is real. She is innocent in all of this. She didn't ask for that gene. She was born with it, and now she has to deal with it.

Being sober and being a parent of a child who drinks is also a double-edged sword. You know exactly how to fix the problem, but you also have to be acutely aware of the reaction you are going to receive if and when you bring it up to your child. The easy reaction is to blow up and scream at her and yell how disappointed you are in her and that she should have known better because of all the shit that you had previously been through. You can ground her for weeks and months and take away her privileges until she has "learned her lesson."

I wish it were that easy.

Kids are going to do what they are going to do. If she is not ready to hear all of my knowledge on alcoholism, then she is not going to pay attention to any of it. As a matter of fact, she might go the opposite way. She might become an expert in hiding her drinking. She might never want to reach out to me when she does want to stop. She might see me as the "enemy." The only reason I know about these reactions is because I have lived it.

Additionally, when you are that young (between fifteen and eighteen years old), it is very difficult to discern what type of drinker you truly are. You feel that "everyone" drinks—and that "everyone" drinks a lot. There is a feeling that all you are doing is following what all of your friends are doing. You do not see drinking as anything unusual or out of the ordinary because you are just following the crowd—herd mentality. The first people who notice you are drinking "out of the ordinary" are typically going to be those who are in your close social circle. And for one of those close crew members to "rat you out" is a major taboo. Your problem drinking can go on and on for quite a while before it needs to be addressed—or before you are forced to address it.

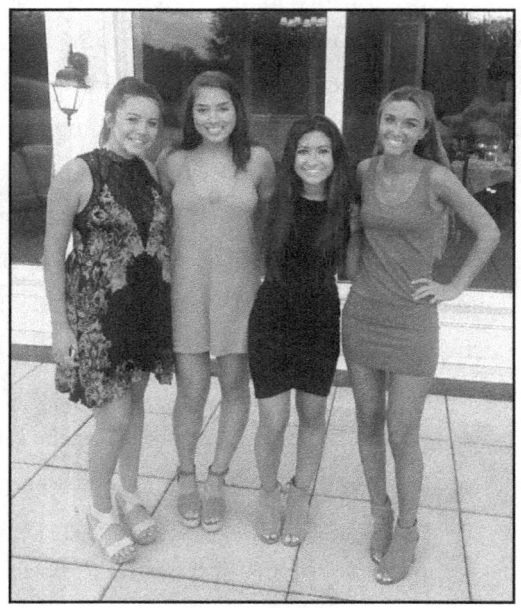

Jill Duerkop, Celeste Rodriguez, my daughter Isabelle, and Molly Paddock having a laugh at the Park Ridge Country Club

THE PARTIES

December 2016

"MY DAD DOESN'T want to come home to see this shit! Everybody, get the fuck out!"

It was December 31, 2016—New Year's Eve. I had organized a small dinner party at the Park Ridge Country Club. It was a nice time with my daughters Sarah and Isabelle, who was seventeen at the time, and another family with their younger kids. We discussed what everyone was doing later that evening. Sarah said she was going to go to a bar/restaurant for the midnight celebration, and Isabelle said she was just going to "lay low"—whatever that meant.

After dinner, I went to a party in my neighborhood and then joined my oldest daughter Sarah at her party at the restaurant, which was not too far away. It was now about 1:30 a.m., and I had had enough of the New Year's Eve crowd. I decided to call it a night. I live on the third floor of a condominium complex and took the elevator to my floor. As I approached my door, I heard very loud noises and just figured that Isabelle had the television turned on very loudly—at high decibel levels.

When I entered my three-bedroom condo, I thought I had stepped into the filming of the 2012 movie *Project X*, about three high school seniors who try to gain popularity by throwing a party nobody would ever forget. I was absolutely flabbergasted. There were at least a hundred kids in my condo!

IT WAS ARMAGEDDON!

There were two DJs in two separate rooms with all of their equipment.

There were people smoking weed and drinking in each one of my bedrooms.

Several kids were smoking cigars like they had just won the NBA championship.

There was an Italian food spread on my kitchen table catered by Zia's Trattoria.

There was even a fucking tarot card reader in my bedroom.

I could not believe my eyes. I was speechless, dazed, and exhausted. Several of Isabelle's friends greeted me with gigantic smiles on their faces. Everyone was drunk and/or high. It was the party of the century. I attempted to look for Isabelle, who was nowhere to be found among the crowd.

One of Isabelle's friends, Kelly, approached me and slurred this gem to me:

"Mr. Arana, don't worry about a thing. Here is a cigar. Please smoke it and relax. I will be over first thing in the morning to help you clean up."

As I was attempting to process the absurdity of what Kelly was telling me, I saw Isabelle. She looked at me and, without hesitation, yelled to the entire crowd:

"My dad doesn't want to come home to see this shit! Everybody, get the fuck out!"

I was amazed that all of her friends actually listened and began to disperse quickly. The DJs needed some assistance carrying their gigantic speakers down three flights of stairs. We had to wrap up the food and give it away to the departing guests. I had to gather all of the beer cans, beer bottles, vodka bottles, and wine bottles and put them in large garbage bags and throw them out. I had to vacuum all of the rooms to remove cigarette ashes, cigar ashes, and blunt ashes from the carpet. I had to put all of the dishes in the dishwasher after pre-rinsing them. I was finally done with the cleanup at about 4 a.m. Whew! It was time to get to bed.

Wait one second. Where was Isabelle? Shit! I had lost her amidst the commotion of the party and the massive cleanup effort. Where had she gone? I looked in every bedroom, closet, and bathroom, and she was nowhere to be found. Please don't tell me she went back out after the party, I thought.

I started to walk the final bag of garbage down the three flights of stairs leading to the first floor when I overheard a faint clanking of glasses. I could barely make out the sound. I proceeded down to the basement level of my building and saw Isabelle curled up sleeping in a fetal position, clutching a champagne glass and hugging the biggest bottle of Grey Goose vodka I had ever seen in my life.

I shook her and asked her what the hell was going on. Her response:

"Oh, hey Dad. I am just waiting for a friend to pick me up. We are going to another party."

Please keep in mind that it was now about 4:15 a.m., and I was exhausted. I responded to Isabelle's brilliant plan with my own plan for her:

"That sounds wonderful, Isabelle. But how about we take you upstairs and you can take a little nap.? As soon as your friend gets

197

here, I will wake you up and you can go to your party. Does that sound good?"

Isabelle: "Dad, that is a great idea!"

Let's just say her friend never showed up and Isabelle slept until 5 p.m. the following afternoon.

Oh, and Kelly never showed up to help me clean up. Shocking.

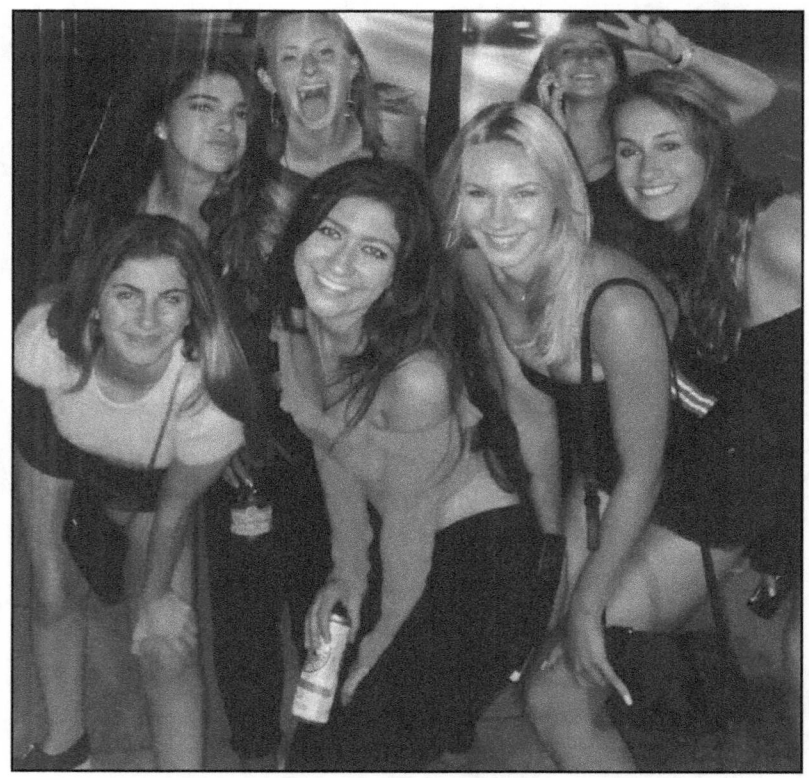

Isabelle enjoying a night out with her camp work friends

Isabelle regularly held "gatherings" with her friends during the summer of 2016 on my outdoor deck, which is on the third floor of my condominium in Chicago's Edison Park neighborhood. This was the summer between her senior year of high school and her freshman year of college. The get-togethers started off innocently enough with a couple of her girlfriends eating pizza and gossiping (or so I thought). I enjoyed it when Isabelle's friends came over because I felt that she would not get into much trouble and I could control her better when she was at home.

The word spread among Isabelle's friends that she was hosting "porch parties," as they were referred to. These gatherings evolved into full-fledged ragers as the summer progressed. I would order pizza and chicken wings and burgers as the crowds started to get larger. These girls became experts at hiding alcohol. Every time I entered the deck, I never saw any alcohol anywhere. Where had they hid it?

My bedroom was far away enough from my deck where I could not really hear much of what was going on. And I did not want to hear anything. Most nights, I just wanted to go to sleep, and I was simply happy that Isabelle was home and that she was safe. In retrospect, I should have supervised those parties more closely. I wasn't that stupid. I cleaned up their mess every morning after the porch parties. The hiding places for the bottles were in very obvious places—like under my barbecue grill.

One day, I received an email from my condo association president requesting an explanation for a letter he had received from my neighbor across the street complaining about the "porch parties." It detailed all kinds of crazy allegations (which I am sure were all true) about loud parties lasting all night and keeping the neighbors up. I was so pissed off. I showed Isabelle the letter, and, of course, she had no idea what the letter was about. She claimed complete innocence regarding the porch parties.

I put an end to the parties. I explained to Isabelle that she was endangering my living situation and that I simply could not have that.

She could no longer have her friends on my porch. I put my foot down. This had started to become embarrassing for me.

Well, the moratorium on the parties lasted for about a week. Everything calmed down temporarily, and then Isabelle and her friends ramped it up again for the remainder of the summer and into the following year. I failed as a parent in that situation. I should have stuck with my ban of the parties. But I suppose the guilt of my alcoholism and the desire to be a "cool" parent prevented me from doing the right thing.

In retrospect, I should have been stern with Isabelle. I should have stuck with the groundings and the punishments and the consequences. I am not sure if this would have changed her behavior, but maybe it would have prevented a few of the incidents that would follow. Perhaps it would have only prolonged the inevitable. Teenagers are going to find a way no matter what. You just have to hope and pray that the life lessons you have instilled in them will eventually kick in before it is too late.

Being divorced is also not an ideal way to raise children. There are always slippages that can occur when you are not making decisions together with your partner on how to raise your children. Thankfully, T. C. and I were on the same page regarding Isabelle and her drinking. The problem was that we were not exactly sure of the measures we had to take in order to help her succeed.

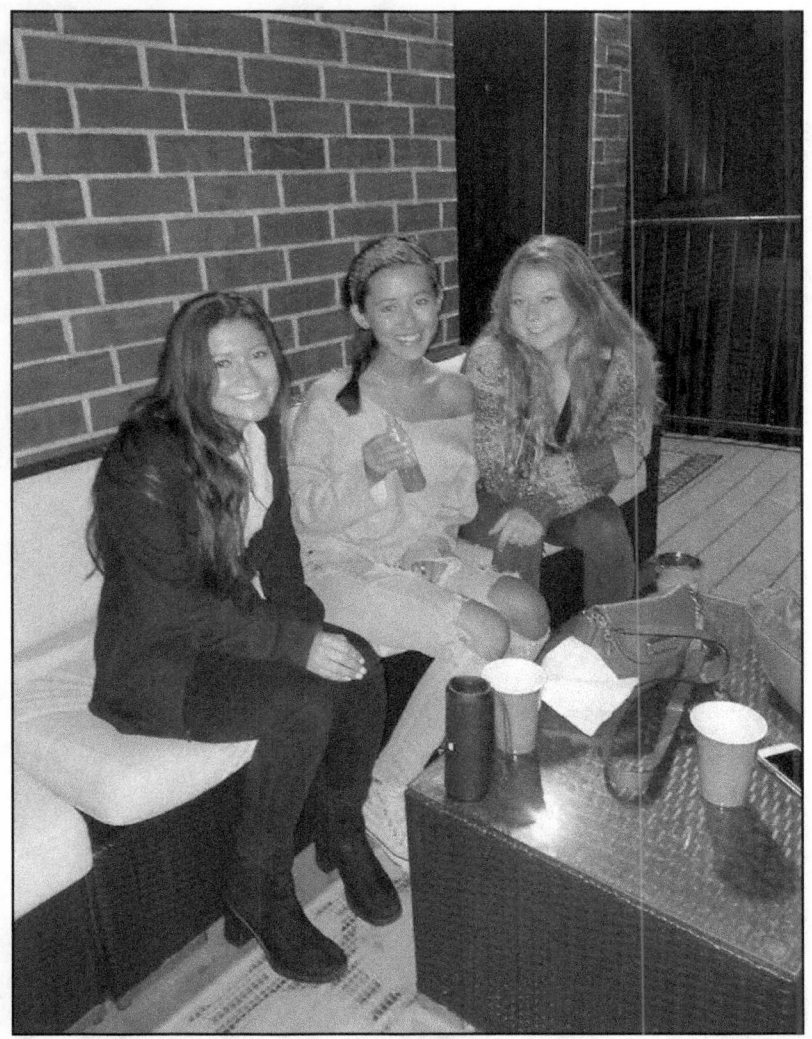

My daughter Isabelle, Kelly Maigler, and Olivia Latreille
looking very innocent—the calm before the storm

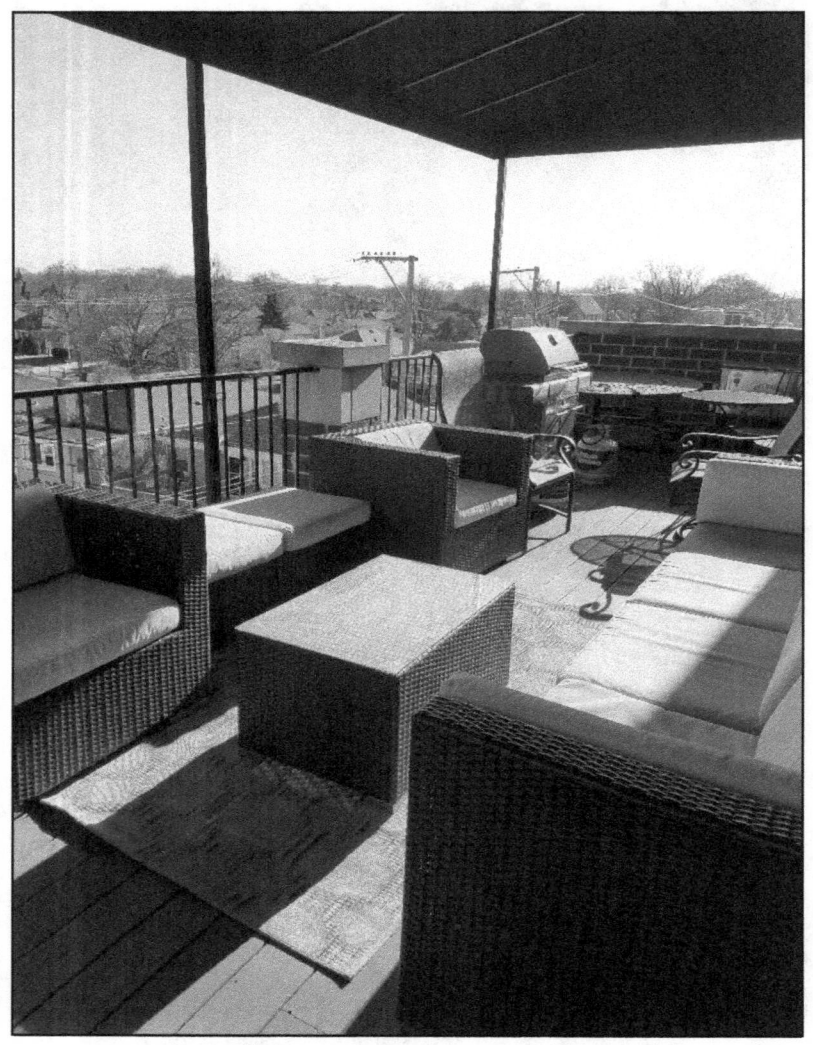

The infamous "porch" where there were many parties

DISASTER IN MADISON

December 2017 to May 2018

ISABELLE WENT AWAY to college at the University of Wisconsin-Madison in Madison, Wisconsin. In her freshman and sophomore year, she was still getting straight As in all of her classes. She had always been a superstar in the classroom. However, her drinking had gone to new levels. We were getting reports of her drinking escapades and her blackouts. As parents, T. C. and I were extremely worried and scared.

There were a few major incidents that happened to Isabelle during her freshman and sophomore year at Wisconsin that I will not get into detail about. They are private and, in Isabelle's words, "her story to tell." Maybe Isabelle will write a book one day describing her journey.

As a parent, I was going through hell. And I knew T. C. was going through hell, too. We felt powerless that we couldn't do anything to prevent her from drinking. When you are a parent of a child who goes away to school, your hands are somewhat tied. You have very little control over what can happen. I wish it had been different. I wish I could have had a camera and microphone on Isabelle twenty-four hours a day, advising her on what she should and should not have been doing.

I cried myself to sleep just thinking about what my daughter was going through on many nights. Everything bad that was happening to her, I wanted it to happen to me instead—that was the amount of guilt I felt. I had given my daughter the alcoholic gene. I had caused this to happen to her. I was the reason she was drinking the way she drank.

Till today, I have an obsession with making sure my cell phone is constantly charged to nearly 100 percent on a daily basis. Originally, it was because I was very worried about my parents, and I wanted to be available in case anything happened to them. But later, my concern about getting a phone call about Isabelle rose to levels that I never thought existed. T. C. and I received phone calls that equated to a "parent's worst nightmare" during Isabelle's freshman and sophomore year. To say I was worried about Isabelle would be the understatement of the century.

Even after my sobriety, this fucking alcoholism continued to kick me in the ass.

What was I going to do to make her understand that this level of drinking was doing her harm? How could I explain to her that she was heading down a path of destruction that I knew the exact directions to?

This was ten times worse than being a drunk myself, because while I could ultimately control my own destiny, this was my daughter. Only she could decide to help herself or continue on this highway to hell.

Isabelle and I would talk on the phone on a regular basis. But I would never get into detail about her drinking. I would just tell her to be careful and to think about what she was doing. I know from experience that if you press a teenager too hard, the opposite effect of what you want to accomplish might occur. I did not want that to happen. I knew Isabelle was aware that her drinking bothered me a lot. I knew that Isabelle read my many Facebook posts about sobriety. I hoped and

I prayed that maybe a little of that would rub off on her. The days of grounding Isabelle for bad behavior were over. She was legally an adult. We could only pray that the values we had instilled in her would be enough for her to weather this storm and make her see a better path.

Nobody is going to listen to anyone unless they experience the negative aspects and consequences that are a result of drinking for themselves—especially if they are teenagers. Drinking inspires a great deal of curiosity in young people. They want to see for themselves what it is all about—and, for the most part, drinking is a lot of fun. Drinking brings people together and makes socializing a lot easier and less awkward. But there is such a fine line between drinking alcohol and abusing alcohol. Sometimes it takes a lifetime of experiences to figure it out.

I felt that Isabelle was in a very bad place. Unfortunately, I knew where this story was headed. I knew exactly where this demon and this disease wanted to take her. However, she never wanted to discuss getting help from me. I would have been the perfect person to go to; I was fifteen years sober at the time. But I understood that the only time a person asks for help is when they want the help. I loved her so much and felt helpless in so many ways.

My strategy was hope, and hope was not a strategy.

THE PHONE CALL

February 22, 2019

ISABELLE AND I have a very close relationship. When she was away at college, we would speak at least four or five times a week. I was extremely worried about what was going to happen to her next. She was drinking and blacking out at an alarming rate. It was just a matter of time before the next Isabelle-related catastrophe would take place. I made sure my cell phone was right next to me while I slept just in case I received a phone call that would require me to make a road trip to Madison in order to save Isabelle from herself.

Isabelle called me on a Sunday night, just like she did on any other night. We talked about how school was going and that she had a couple of tests coming up the following week that she had to study for. Once again, we didn't bring up her drinking. She knew my history with alcoholism and that her drinking bothered and worried me tremendously, while I was aware that if I became too angry at her, I ran the the risk of alienating and losing her forever.

Usually, Isabelle ended every phone call with "Love you." But this time, Isabelle wrapped up our conversation by telling me this:

"Oh, by the way, Dad, did you know that I haven't had a drink in six weeks? I thought you would like that."

Isabelle mentioned how she had had a conversation with her doctor who had suggested that she quit drinking. I told Isabelle how great that was. I congratulated her and told her how proud I was of her, and we hung up.

But in reality, I was doing jumping jacks in my head.

She hadn't had a drink in six weeks? Was she kidding me? I was literally leaping out of my skin in happiness. I could not believe what I had just heard.

It made total sense because I had not had to deal with any Isabelle problems during that time frame. Could she keep it up? Had the light bulb finally gone on in her head? This was the best news that I could have possibly imagined. As a parent, this was better than any report card she could have gotten. I was in tears that night—of happiness. Could this be the beginning of a new life for her? I didn't want to get my hopes up too high because I know how hard (nearly impossible) it is for young people to attain sobriety.

I prayed to God that she would keep it up.

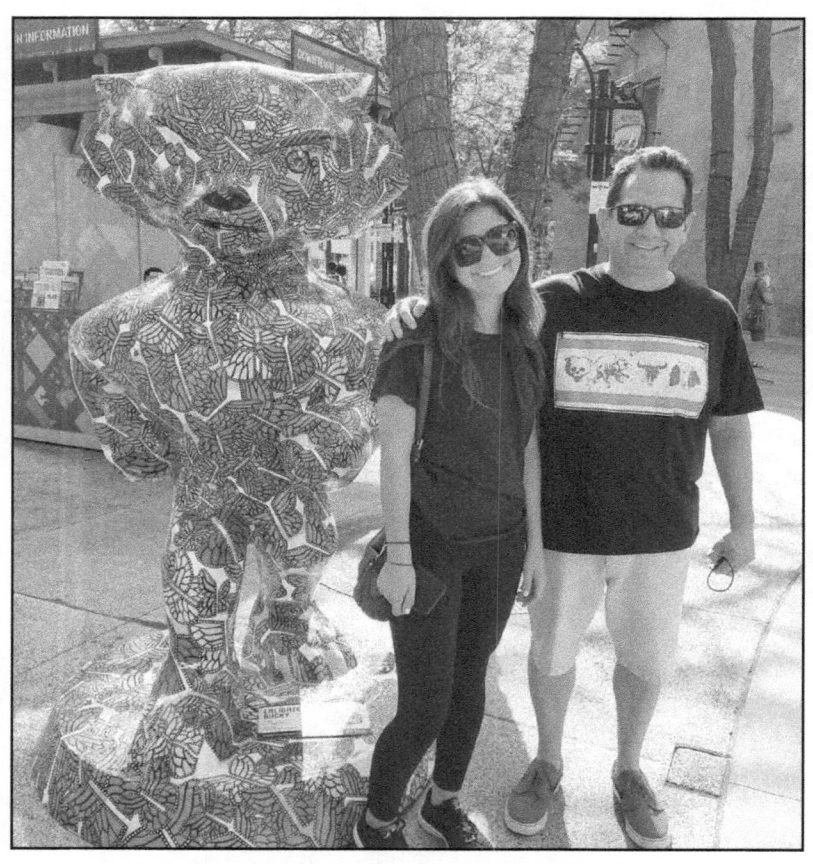

Isabelle and I at the University of Wisconsin-Madison.

ISABELLE'S JOURNEY TOWARD HER FIRST YEAR OF SOBRIETY

January 11, 2019, to the Present

THE FOLLOWING POSTS and pictures were taken chronologically from my Facebook posts throughout Isabelle's journey toward her first year of sobriety. One of my main mantras in remaining sober is to make a big deal about your sobriety. You become accountable to your friends and family and, most importantly, yourself. I wanted to support Isabelle every step of the way through her daily struggles. I didn't want to push too hard, either. Sobriety is such a personal struggle that everyone finds their own unique way.

APRIL 21, 2019

I know somebody who is 100 days sober today! Guess what? It is a gigantic deal! Congratulations! What a fucking feeling! There are so many milestones in sobriety. I remember my 100-day mark like it was yesterday. It was the first time that I actually thought I could beat this thing. I am so happy for you and so proud of you. The average person has no idea how difficult this accomplishment is. The average person can go about a week or so and feel great, and then all of a sudden—BOOM! Something happens, usually life happens, and the sobriety doesn't last. It's okay, though. Keep picking yourself up and try again. You can do it. 100 days! 2,400 hours! 144,000 minutes! 8,640,000 seconds! You did not drink! You were strong enough not to do it! You made a decision that might possibly save your life! Let me ask you a question, mystery 100-day person: Has your life become better or worse in these last 100 days? I think I have a pretty good idea of the answer. **Congrats** and keep up the good work! I am so fucking happy for you! Please comment and give this person some positive feedback. Hoppy Easter!

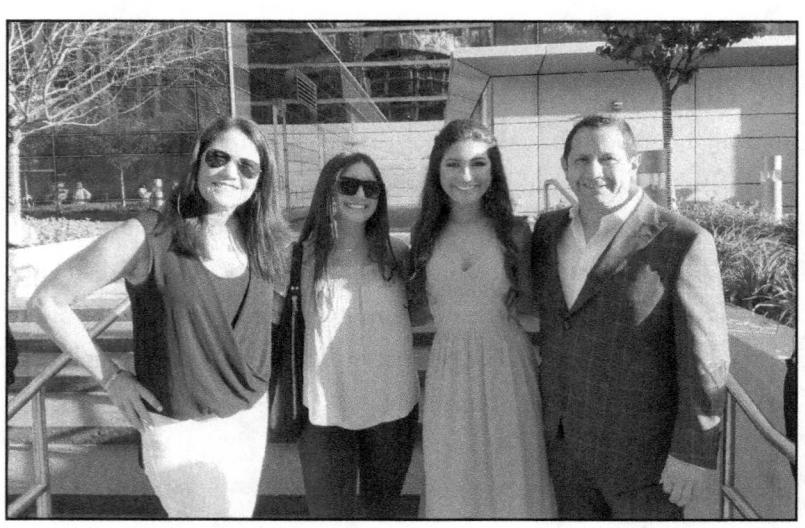

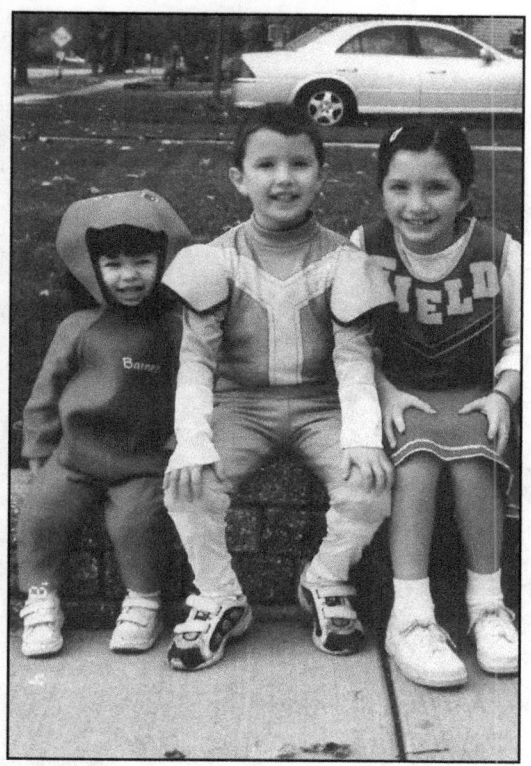

MAY 17, 2019

We celebrated my daughter Isabelle Arana's 125th day of sobriety last night. Once again, she received straight As at the University of Wisconsin-Madison, but that REALLY takes a back seat to this accomplishment. We all love you and support you and wish you continued success! #isabellestrong #soberaf #alcoholism #alcoholic #recovery #sobriety #125days

(Note: The celebration dinner took place at Ceviche Peruvian Seafood & Steakhouse at 2554 W. Diversey in Chicago.)

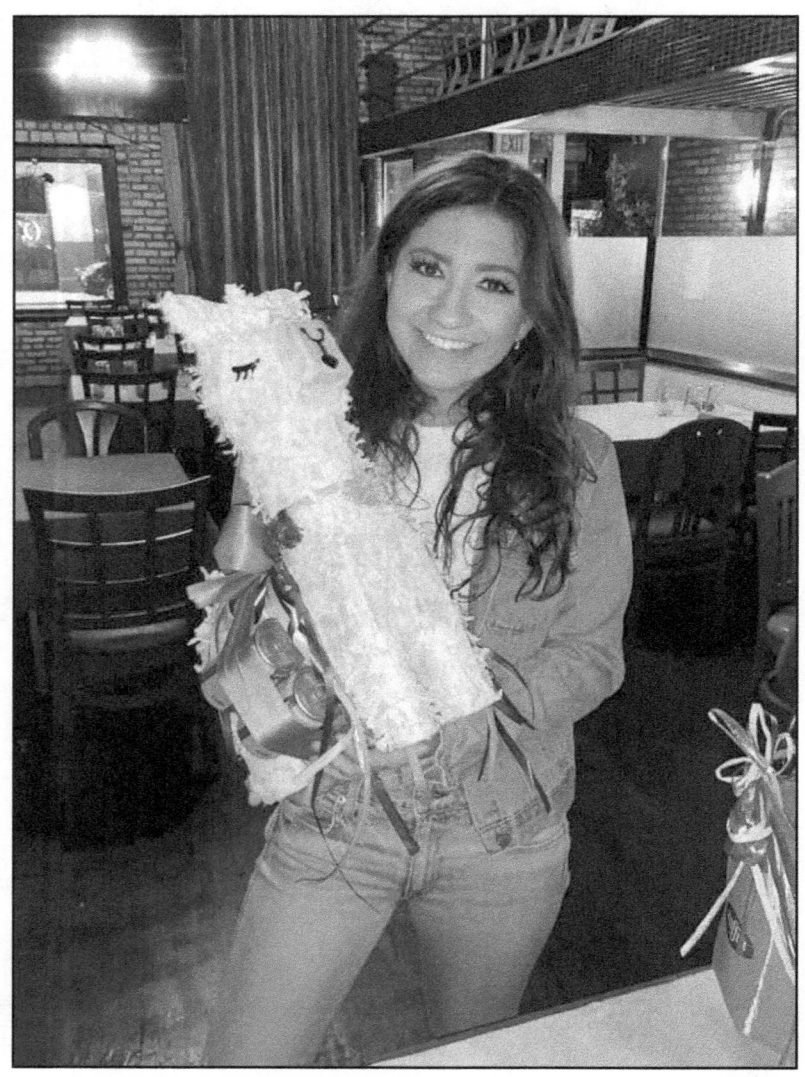

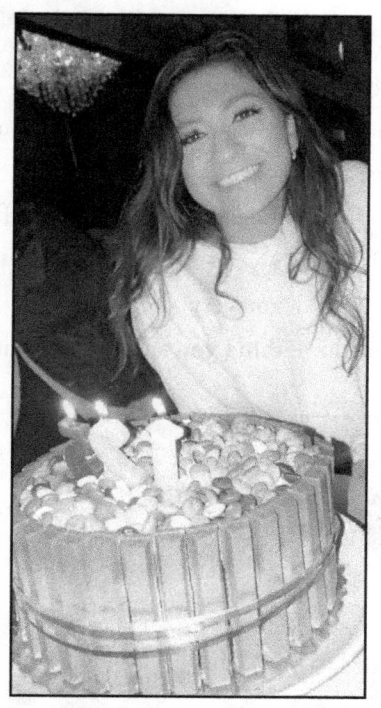

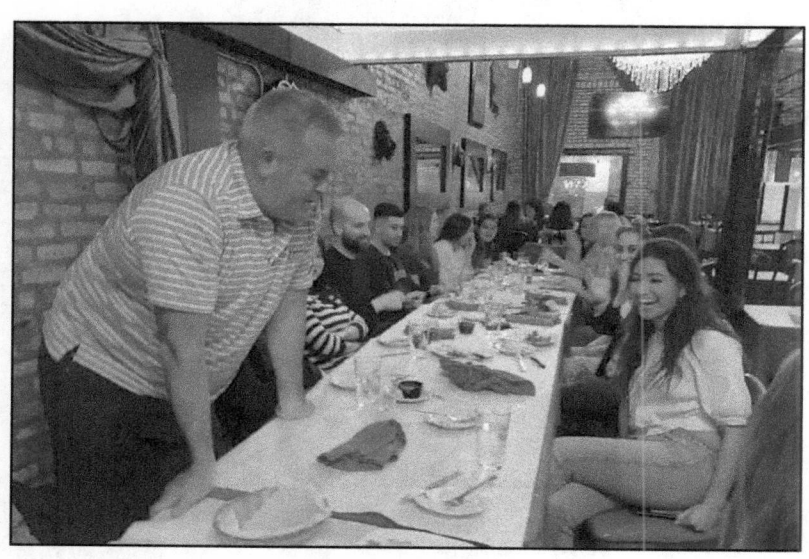

JUNE 3, 2019

Just in case anybody is wondering, Isabelle Arana is 143 days sober today! Yes, it is a major deal. Reach out and congratulate her! Being an alcoholic is not a disease that is hidden away anymore. Be proud of her! It is okay to talk about it! She is extremely proud of it. Does anybody realize how hard it is for a 19-year-old to have 143 days of sobriety? Big deal! Congrats, Isabelle! I am very proud of you. Being sober is an accomplishment, not something you should be ashamed of. #soberAF

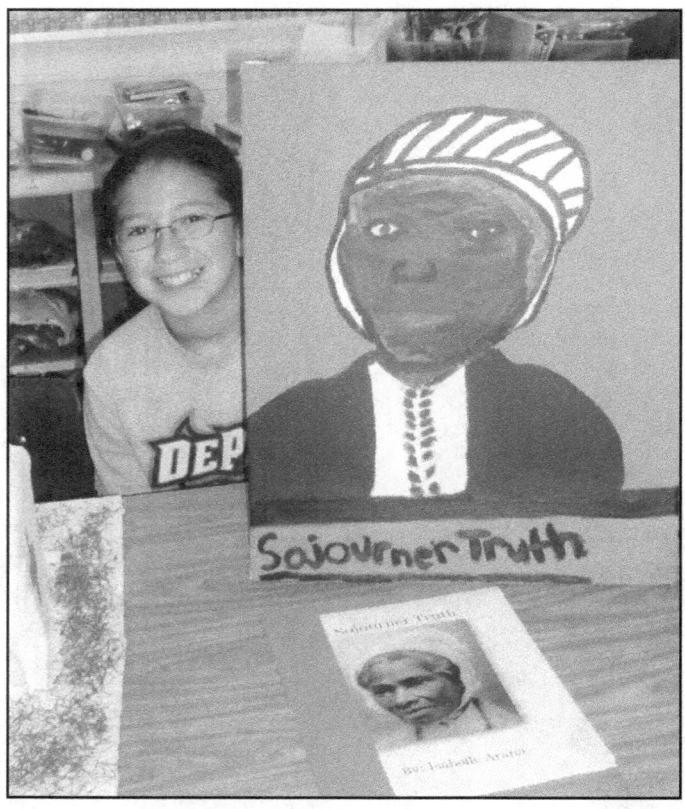

JUNE 22, 2019

Wait a second! Wait a second! Can you say 162 days sober for Isabelle Arana? Does anybody know how hard this is for a 19-year-old kid? This is summer in Chicago. This is drinking every fucking night when you are this age. This is bars, clubs, rooftops, house parties, porch parties, and ball games. She is staying strong! She is a beast! I truly believe you celebrate this kind of thing! Alcoholism is out of the closest! Be proud of your sobriety! Do the next right thing! If you think you have a problem and you are a young kid or an adult, do not despair. There is hope. Get help. Life is too great to live it in shame. Proud alcoholic father! #soberaf #isabellestrong

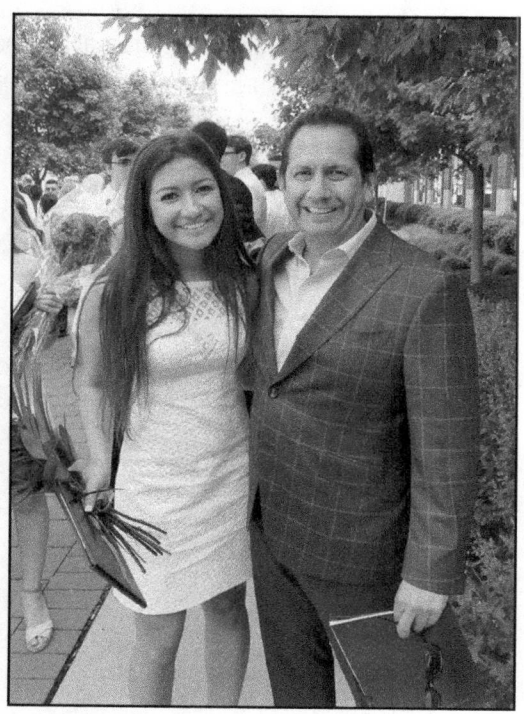

JULY 11, 2019

Isabelle Arana is 6 months sober today! This is a huge deal. This is a reason to celebrate! What an accomplishment! Please reach out to her and congratulate her today. If you are a young person, you know how hard this is. You know that it is a hard thing to even think about, much less do. This is my greatest source of pride for Isabelle Arana. Yes, the straight As, the volunteer work at homeless shelters, the house building in Peru, the tutoring of inner city youth are all important, but 6 months sober for a 19-year-old kid? This is amazing! Congratulations, Isabelle Arana! I wish you nothing but continued success, and it is okay to fail. I will be here to pick you up. I love you.

[**Note:** The dinner celebration and pictures were, again, at Ceviche Peruvian Seafood & Steakhouse at 2554 W. Diversey Ave. in Chicago, Illinois.]

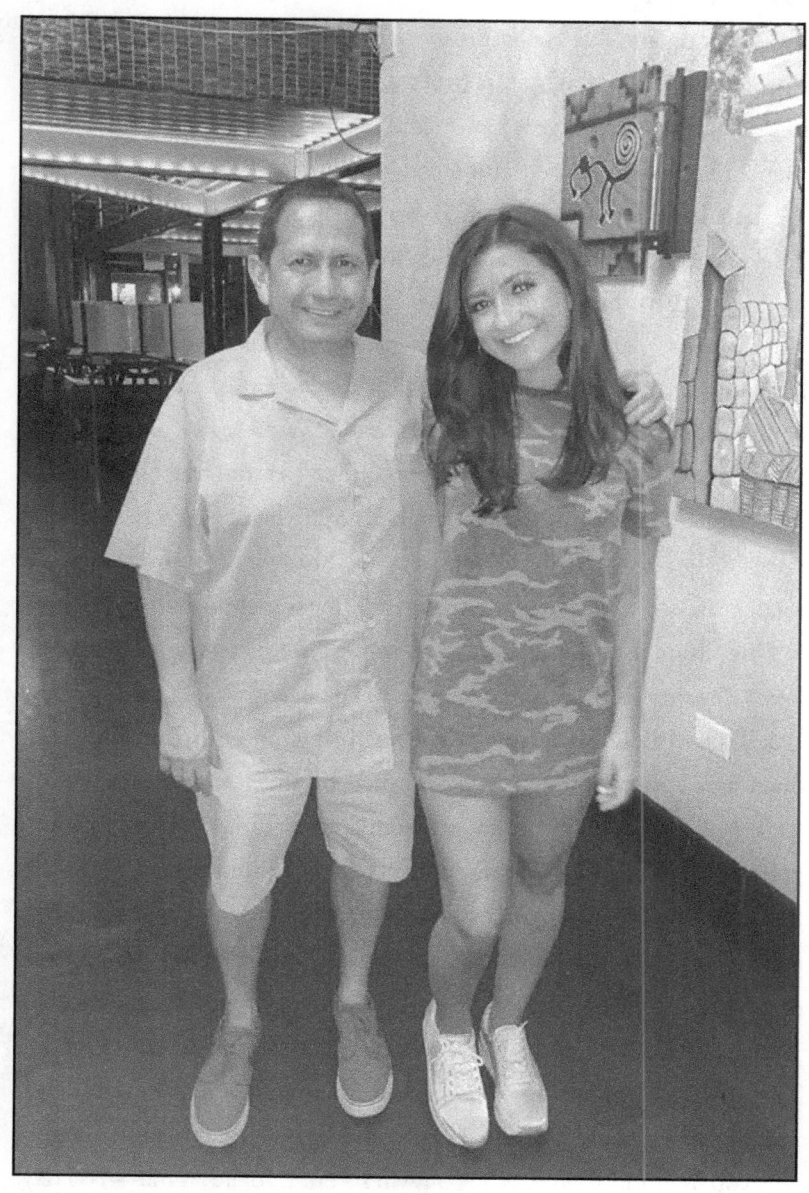

JULY 15, 2019

I was driving an Uber on Saturday night, and it was about 2 a.m. when I picked up two young adults (male and female) near the Emerald Isle in Edison Park. They were hammered. So, naturally, I started to talk to them. The male told me that he had gone to St. Pat's High School and the female told me that she had gone to Resurrection High School. They were both in college, and they were enjoying a summer night out. I thanked them for taking an Uber and for not drinking and driving. They were very drunk but extremely friendly people. We started talking about mutual friends, and then I asked them if they might know my daughter, Isabelle Arana. The female said, "Wait a second, isn't that the girl who is 6 months sober? I read about her on Facebook. She is incredible!" My world literally stopped right there. She did not know Isabelle, but she had heard of Isabelle through the power of social media. Isabelle had made a difference in somebody's life! She was talking about Isabelle like she was some type of young people's folk hero. She went on and on about how her friends were talking about Isabelle and how brave she was about trying to get sober and being open and honest about it. I was floored by this conversation. This is what I have been trying to get across to people, especially young people. But I am too fucking old for people to understand and really listen to. But a young person, like Isabelle, can really make a difference to other young people. Why would a young person listen to an older person? Typically, drinking is a trial and error experience for young people. The trial is that you go out and get fucked up—a lot. The error is that your life gets fucked up after you drink—a lot. It is actually very simple. But if a 19-year-old kid who has been through it tells you about it, then maybe you will listen. Isabelle Arana—185 days sober today.

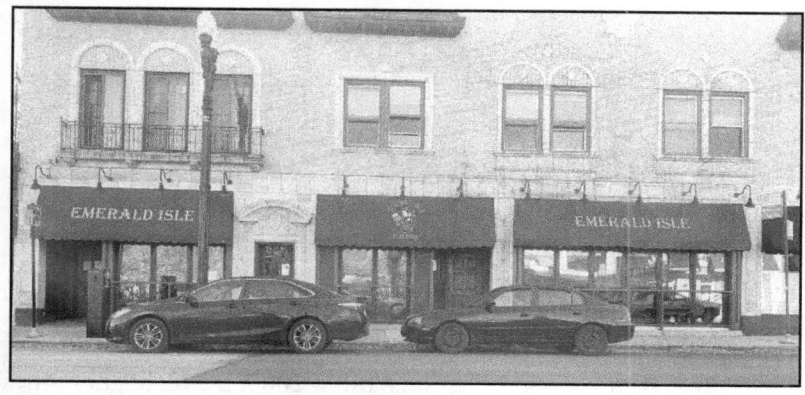

AUGUST 14, 2019

When I was a teenager, I was fully aware that I did not drink like everybody else. Every time that I drank, I wanted to get black-out drunk. I had no clue what "casual" drinking meant. I didn't even like the taste of alcohol. I just loved what it did to me. I loved the euphoria that it created inside of my mind and body. I felt like I was invincible. But every now and then in my late teens, I started to feel bad about my drinking, I guess you could call it guilt. I knew deep down that this was not the right way to act and that it was not good for me. I made attempts to stop. I actually thought that one week of not drinking was a major accomplishment. If I could go one week without it then I really did not have a problem, right? It was a major mind fuck. You know you are not going to stop completely—I mean, why should you? So you just take a few days off, and then you convince yourself that you are like everybody else and that you can continue to drink as much as you want or as much as your body can possibly handle. I thought it wasn't affecting my life much. I was still getting straight As at DePaul University, and I was on a pretty good path in life. I would be able to control this small drinking problem once I got older. Everybody drinks as teenagers and in their early twenties. Maybe I got carried away just a little (well, actually a lot) more than my friends. As a teenager, there were parties every weekend. If you stopped drinking for the week, that meant you missed at least two days of major fun. I really could not stop drinking for more than a week. It was a social impossibility. By this time in my drinking career, I had already been arrested for my drinking, I had gone to the hospital a few times for my drinking, and I had lost a job due to my drinking. In other words, I was fine and there was no reason to stop (sarcasm). Fast forward to 2005: the highlight of my day was walking my 5-year-old daughter Isabelle to Field School, holding her little hand and talking to her for that block and a half. It was my first year of sobriety, and the little things like that make you appreciate what you have in life. It makes you appreciate what is truly important. Fast forward to 2019: Isabelle Arana, 213 days sober today. That is about 28 weekends in case your math is bad. She is a better man than me.

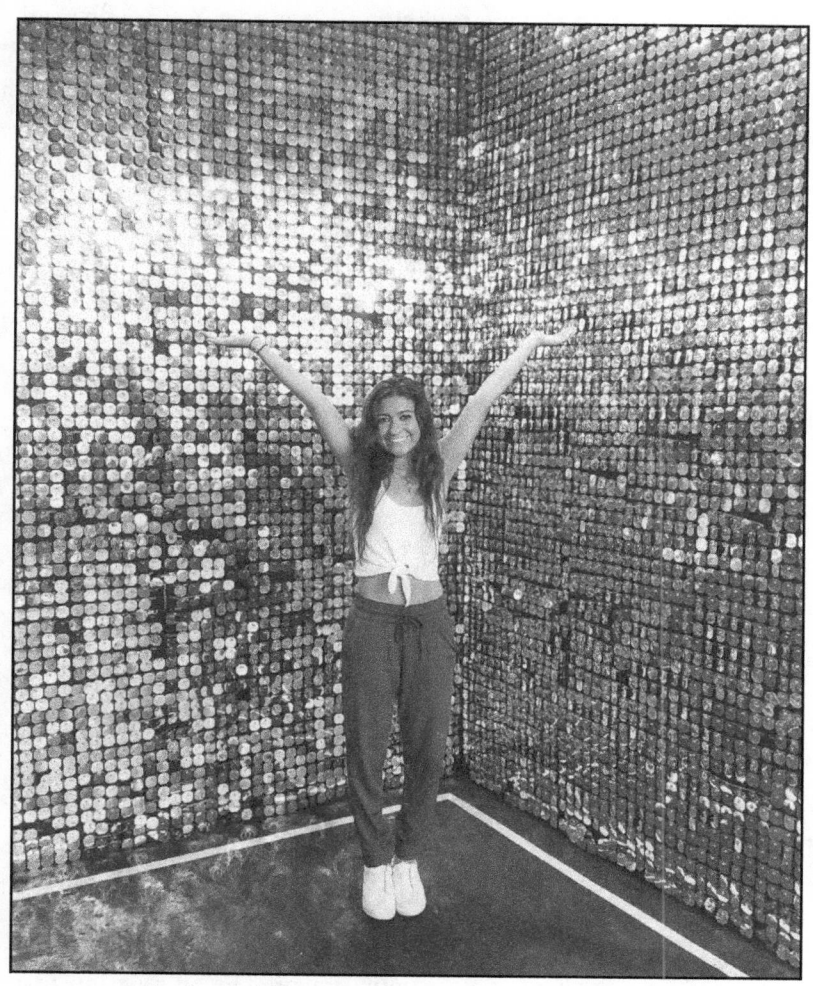

SEPTEMBER 21, 2019

This is an open letter to all young alcoholics. If you are not a young alcoholic, please stop fucking reading this right now. You are fine and you do not need any of my advice. I would define an "alcoholic" as somebody who has continually gotten themselves into problems (minor and/or major) due to their drinking. In other words, you have gotten caught. Your drinking has put you in situations that you would not be in had you been sober. It is a very simple definition. Again, if you do not meet this definition, then you should not read this because you are fine. Let me guess: you are still reading.

Hypothetically speaking, let us assume that you have 253 days of sobriety, which is a major accomplishment—that is over 8 months for those of you who are mathematically challenged. Things are going great, right?

Unfortunately, that little voice in the back of your mind is saying, "Fuck, everybody else is having fun and drinking, and I can't drink. I have this fucking sobriety that I have to maintain. I think I have proven a point—253 days is good enough. I have proven that I can stop. Maybe if I have one drink, I can feel normal again and be part of the crowd. I can fit in again and not have to feel weird. Nobody will know. I can handle it. One drink is not going to kill me. Nobody knows what I am going through. This is so hard. I am 19 years old! This is not fair. Why is this happening to me? Why can't I be normal like everybody else?" These are legitimate concerns that I have some answers to. First of all, 253 days is a fantastic accomplishment! The only person that you have to prove a point to is yourself. Nobody else gives a shit—and I mean nobody. This is your life. You are the only person who matters in this journey. If you think having one drink will make you feel "normal" again, you have another thing coming for you. One drink today becomes five drinks next week. Your mind can convince yourself of anything. Your mind convinced you to stop for 253 days as well—remember that. Nobody will know? Bullshit. You will know, and you are the only person who matters. You can handle it? Let's see . . . I have a track record that can prove otherwise.

I believe that this is hard. And, yes, you are only 19 years old, and no, it is not fair. Alcoholism is a disease. You have the disease. There are a lot of others who have the disease. There are people you can talk to and meetings that you can attend to surround yourself with people who can help make you feel better. And I can promise you one thing: 254 days will feel a lot better than 0 days.

STAY STRONG, ISABELLE.

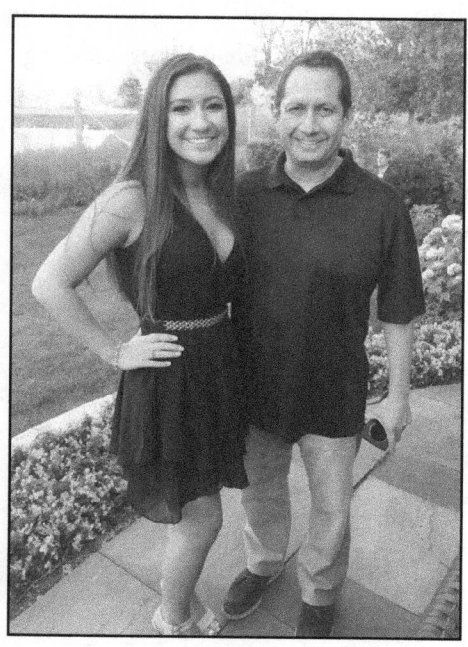

OCTOBER 2, 2019

My daughter Isabelle Arana is 264 days sober today. She is an alcoholic. She is 19 years old. She is a college student. It is okay to call somebody an alcoholic. It is a disease. Do you have the balls to admit that you are an alcoholic? Not too many people have that type of honesty and strength to admit such a thing. Don't worry, I have her permission to call her an alcoholic. It is not a big deal to her. She hopes to bring awareness to young people who also have this disease and to show them that it is okay to admit it. It is okay to go to AA meetings. It is okay not to drink at a party. It is okay to be the only one who is not drunk at a tailgate party. It is okay not to pregame. She can still be at all of these events and have fun. It is okay. It is okay. Don't worry, it is okay. You are not an outsider. You are not weird. Nobody is going to talk about you because nobody gives a shit. Help yourself by saving your life.

264 days sober today. I love you and keep up the good work. I am counting. And it is okay to fail. I can start counting again starting at day one.

Please congratulate her. This is not an easy thing to accomplish, especially at 19 years old.

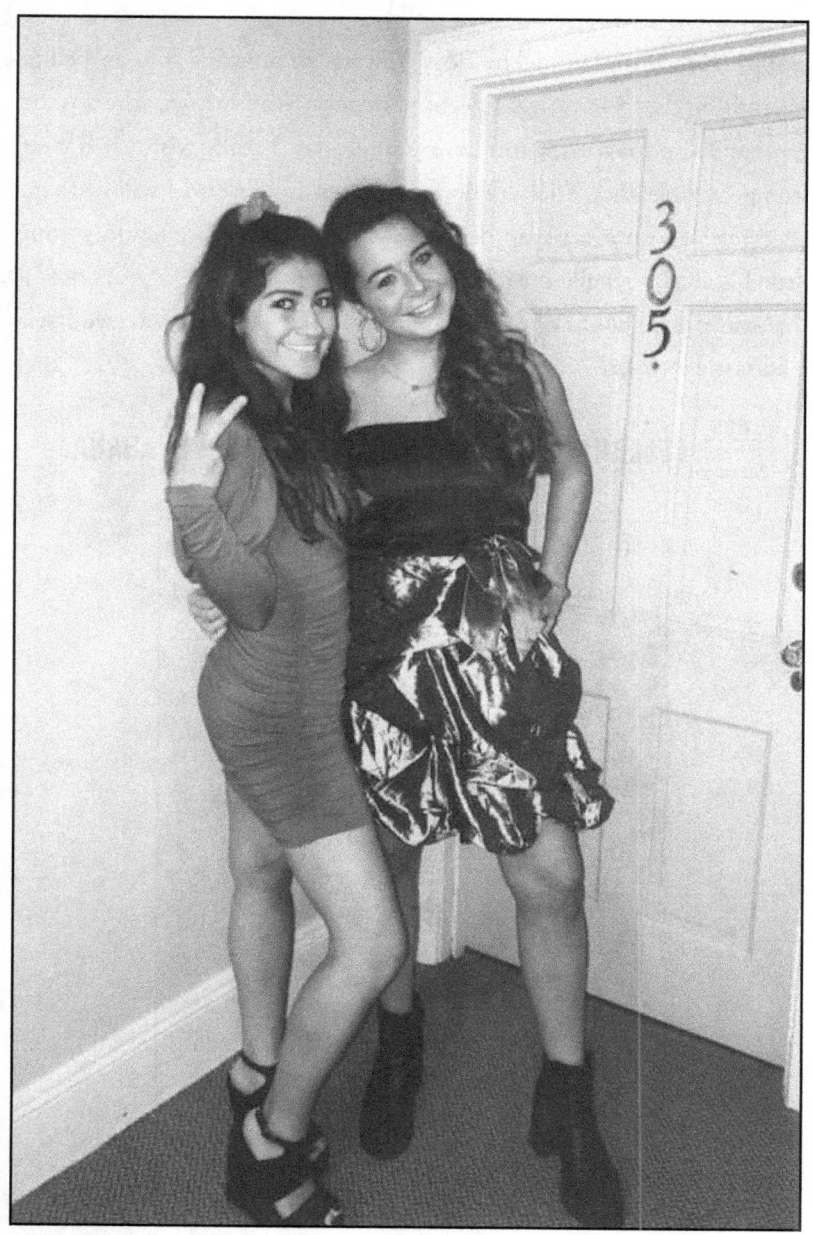

OCTOBER 5, 2019

Happy 20th birthday to The Boss! You are an amazing human being. Everything that you do, you do to perfection. You inspire others to be great and you make me proud every single day. I really wish I had your strength sometimes. You will do great things in life, and I will be there cheering you on every step of the way. I still remember holding your little hand as we walked to Field School when you were 5 years old— that was the highlight of my day. I love you so much and have yourself a fantastic day. #267

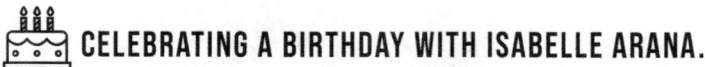 **CELEBRATING A BIRTHDAY WITH ISABELLE ARANA.**

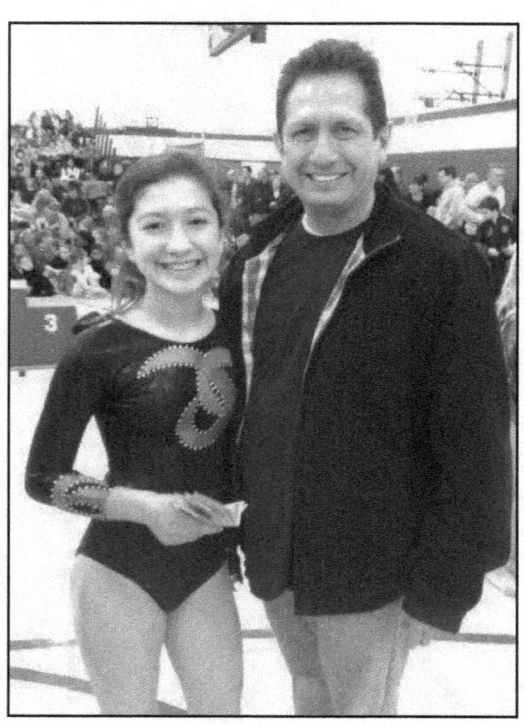

NOVEMBER 8, 2019

Quick shout-out to my amazing daughter Isabelle Arana who is celebrating 300 days of sobriety today! She is at the University of Wisconsin-Madison, and she is receiving straight As in all of her courses. She is planning on attending law school. and there is nothing but sunshine ahead in her life. Almost 10 months of not touching a drink! As the kids say: bet you can't steal this status! We talk every single day about how great it is to be sober. No, every day is not perfect because sobriety does not solve the problems in your life. However, the problems do not get any worse. Imagine being 20 years old and having all of the pressures that a junior in college has, as well as belonging to a sorority and being a social butterfly. This is not an easy feat. If you are a college or high school student, or better yet, if you are a parent of a college or high school student, you know exactly what I am talking about. Congratulations, Isabelle! You are a true inspiration to a lot of people out there! I love you, and, please, always remember: it is okay to fail. It is not the end of the world. You just pick yourself up and start counting again. Here's to 300 days!! Please reach out to her and let her know how great this accomplishment truly is!! #soberaf #isabellestrong

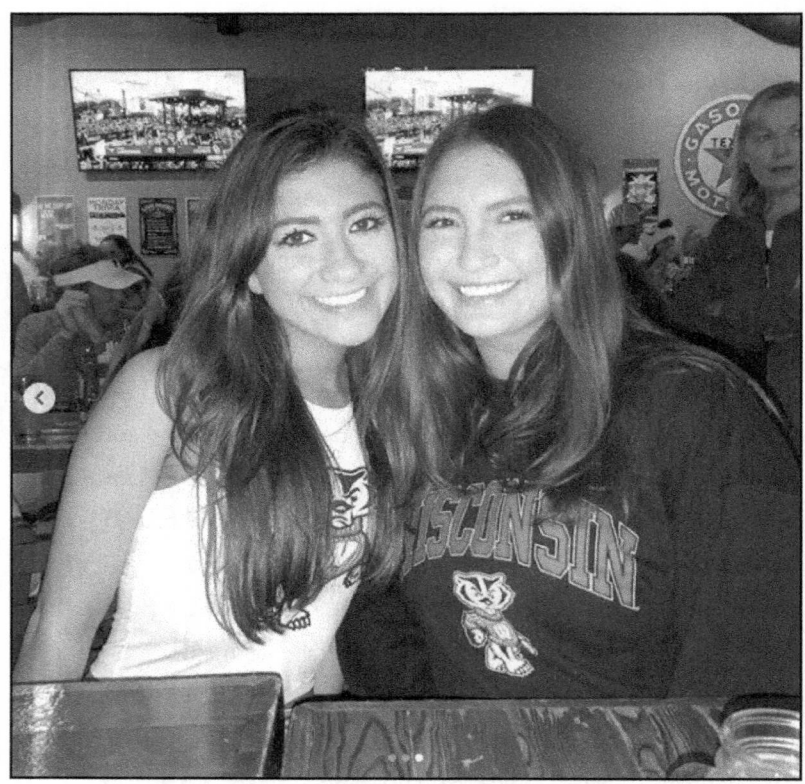

DECEMBER 6, 2019

This is what 329 days of sobriety looks like. It is not glamorous. There are no pics of how fucked up you are at a bar or club. It is about living life. The problems in life are definitely still there, but they sure as fuck are not getting worse. Congratulations, Boss. One day at a time. #isabellestrong #noteasy

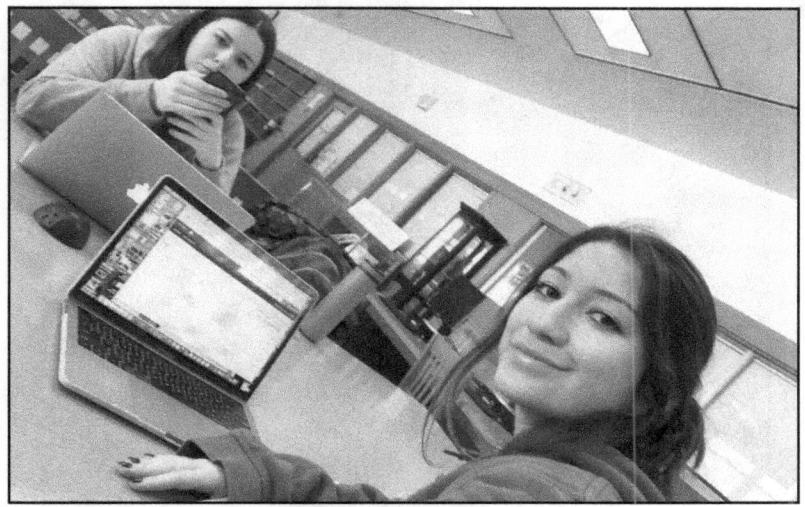

DECEMBER 11, 2019

I know somebody who is 11 months sober today. The people who you least think can do it are the ones who are most likely to succeed. Why? They get sick and tired of being sick and tired. Congratulations, Isabelle Arana. You are a true inspiration to young people and to everybody! Keep up the great work. And it is okay to fail. You just get right back up and try again. I love you.

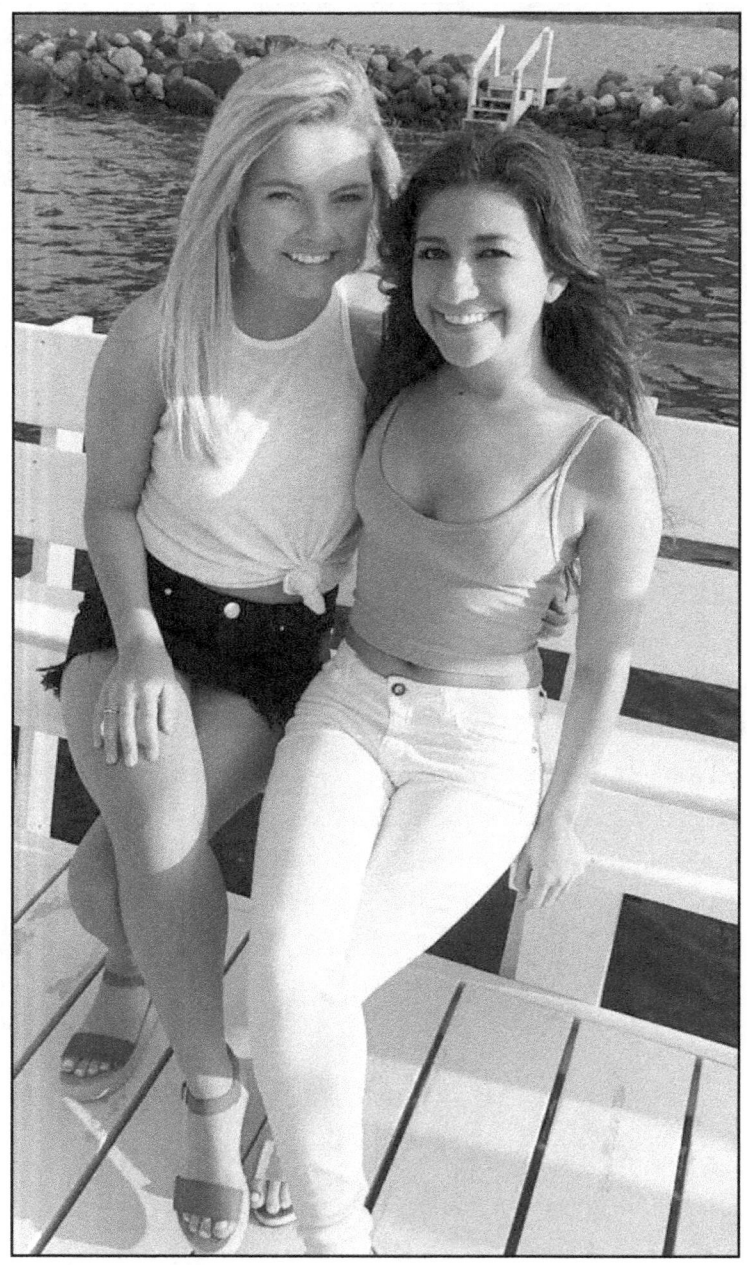

JANUARY 11, 2020

I simply could not wait to write this post. At midnight tonight, my daughter Isabelle Arana will be sober for one year. She is 20 years old. She is 20 years old. She is 20 years old. I think young people can truly understand the magnitude of this achievement. I know people who think they have been drinking too much, and who feel guilty about it and then "take it easy" for a couple of weeks just to shake the cobwebs off and refocus on life. Some people actually do a "dry month" where they are very serious about being sober for a month but then, inevitably, start back up right where they left off without missing a beat.

To be this young and have a year of sobriety is simply amazing. This should be the peak of her drinking career. This is college. This is frat parties and sorority parties. This is major bashes in your hometown when you are home from college. This is having a crew of friends who are no strangers to drinking.

DRINKING is at the epicenter of the life of many young people.

DRINKING makes it easier for you to deal with your parents.

DRINKING makes it easier for you to deal with someone you like, especially when they don't like you.

DRINKING makes it easier to deal with not getting good grades at school.

DRINKING makes it easier to deal with not having enough friends.

DRINKING makes it easier to deal with loneliness.

DRINKING makes it easy to blow off steam after finals week.

DRINKING makes it more fun to go out to dinner.

DRINKING makes you more social at parties.

DRINKING makes sporting events more fun.

DRINKING makes it easier to deal with boredom.

DRINKING is life.

Then, **DRINKING** fucks up your life.

DRINKING puts you in situations that you would never be in.

DRINKING makes your parents worry about you on a nightly basis.

DRINKING makes you depressed and makes you not the person you really are and want to be.

DRINKING causes conflicts with the people who love you and who would do anything to help you.

Isabelle had a scheduled checkup with her doctor about a year ago. Everything checked out great for her physically. But when she was about to leave, the doctor told Isabelle, "Well, you know that you're an alcoholic, right?"

Isabelle has the same doctor as her mom, and her mom had filled the doctor in on Isabelle's life and her drinking episodes and consequences—which were numerous. Isabelle responded with nervous laughter and said, "Wait . . . what?"

(Sidenote: I have noticed that "Wait . . . what?" is really young-people code for "Yes, I have been caught, and please give me a couple of moments so I can formulate a sentence to get myself out of this mess that I have caused.")

Isabelle added, "What are you talking about? I'm so confused." (More classic filler replies that young people often use.) The doctor continued, "Yes, you are an alcoholic. If you continue on this path, you will die. I hope you are aware of this. You need to stop drinking completely." Isabelle just thanked her and left the room.

What does this doctor know about my life? Isabelle thought. How dare her speak to me in that fashion? She doesn't know me. She doesn't know what I have been through. Fuck her.

Isabelle called me a few weeks later from the library at college. We talked like we usually do, and she casually added, "Dad, you know that I haven't drank in 6 weeks?" I responded with, "Wow, that is great, Isabelle! I am so happy for you!" She told me the story of her doctor's appointment and what the doctor had told her about her being an alcoholic. I tried to act composed and tried to process what she had just told me. She hadn't drank in 6 weeks? I was doing jumping jacks in my head! No wonder I hadn't gotten any late-night phone calls for the last month and a half! I was cautiously optimistic that, maybe, she finally got it. I had prayed so long for this day.

I would subsequently get texts from her periodically that would just say, "2 months" or "3 months." I used to count the days, even the hours, when I was getting sober. Isabelle likes to count the months. It's all the same shit. We are both scorekeepers—whatever works to keep you sober.

We had a big dinner for Isabelle for her 125 days of being sober. Her friends showed up and made speeches. Isabelle seemed very proud of herself, and her friends were extremely supportive. The next milestone was her 6-month sobriety dinner. Wow, she was really serious now. Six months of being sober for a 20-year-old is unheard of. Maybe she could do it. More text message followed: "8 months," "10 months," "11 months" . . . . Holy fuck! She was going to make it!

We are in the homestretch. One more day! ONE YEAR of sobriety!! What an accomplishment! This is a final exam that you will take every day of your life. This is a final exam that you have been studying for your whole life. This is a final exam that you can help other people study for. This is a final exam that you can fail at, and this is a final exam that you can retake—and you can still get an A in the class.

> *I love you, Isabelle, with all of my heart, and I know that you are on the path to success in life. I am such a proud dad right now—you have no idea. This is my Super Bowl win. Here's to continued success with your sobriety, and if you slip up, it is okay. It is not the end of the world. You just pick yourself up, and you try again.*

I KNEW I WOULD LOVE WRITING THIS POST.

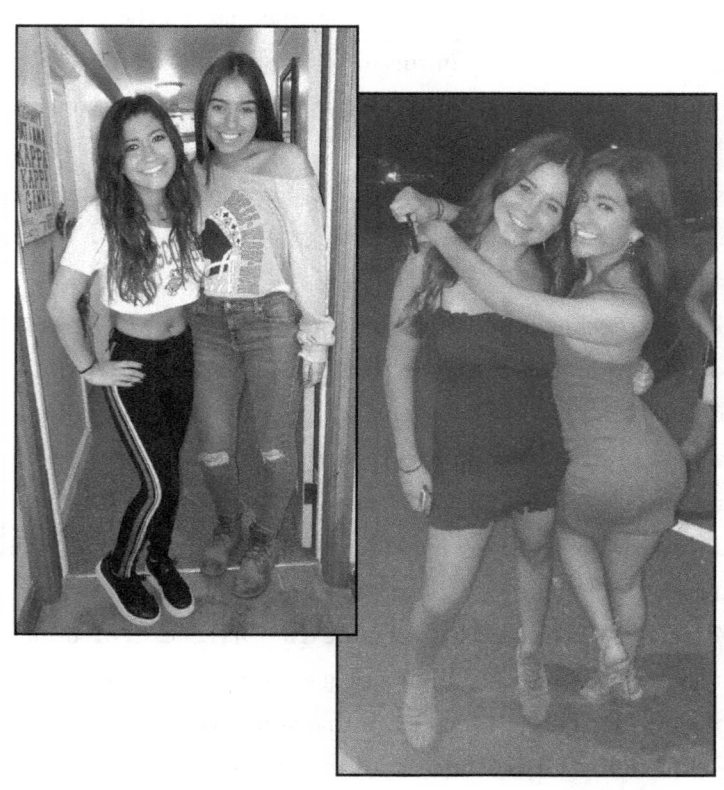

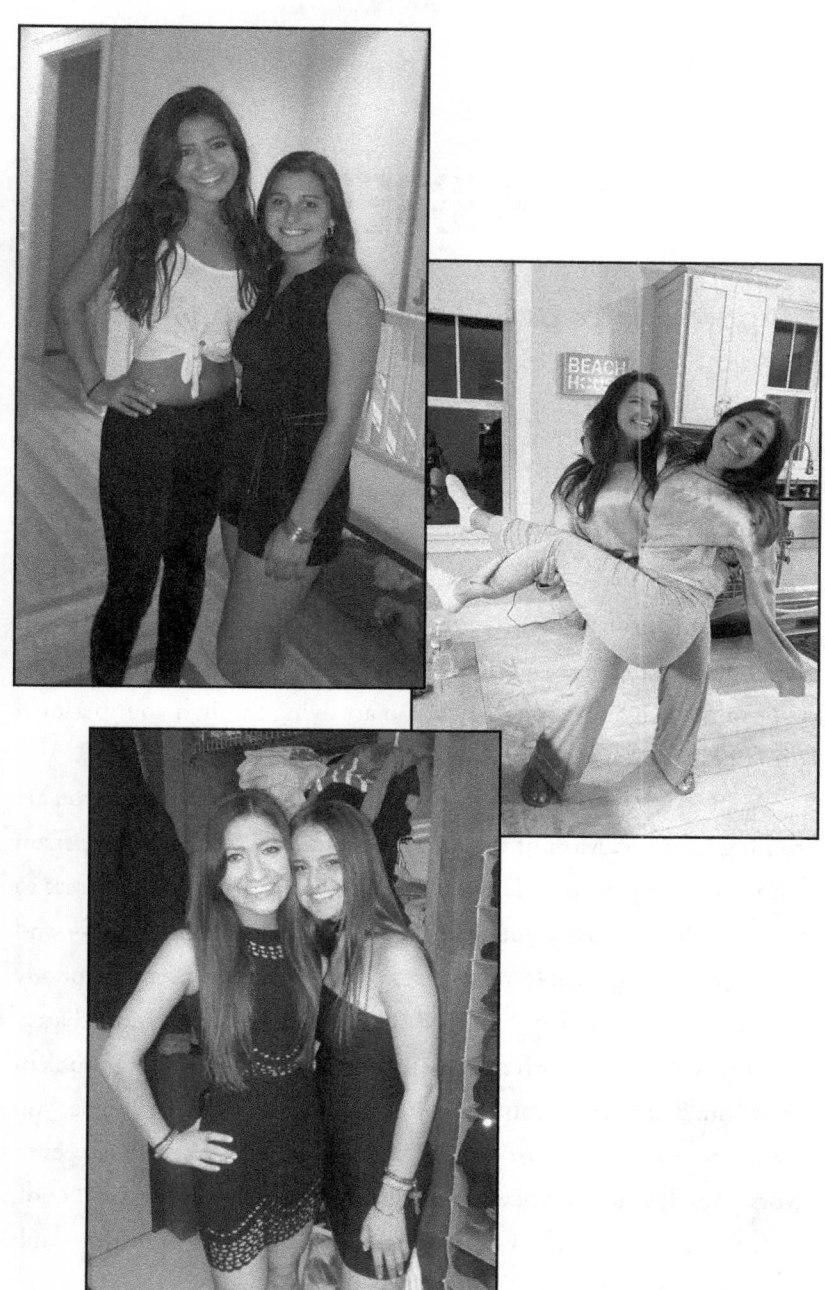

REGRETS

Approximate Date: My Entire Drinking Career

MY SISTER, VIRGINIA, was crying and pleading with me to stop drinking, insisting that I was hurting myself and hurting my parents tremendously. I was eighteen or nineteen years old at the time. I had gotten home from yet another night out with the boys. It was a typical night of drinking beer and doing shots at someone's house or garage or alley in the neighborhood. When you are living through your personal drinking, you really don't think much of it.

People constantly tell you that you should slow down or that you are ruining your life. Most of the time, the solution is to avoid the person who is telling you that. The funny thing is that the people closest to you, which are usually your family, are the first to recognize it—and they are the first people to receive a "fuck you" from you. Nobody wants to hear that they have a drinking problem. You immediately point to someone else who you perceive has a worse drinking problem than you. That makes you feel better for a while, until, of course, you are worse than that person—and then you find someone else even worse. You love to see a person who is more fucked up than you. "Look at Joel! Look how fucked up he is! At least I didn't [fill in the blank with anything fucked up]."

I have such tremendous regret in disappointing my parents and my sister. We had the best family—and still do. I was such an arrogant asshole. I didn't care about anyone but myself. I would take every opportunity I could to leave my family in order to satisfy my alcohol cravings. My parents were the nicest people in the world. They didn't deserve what I put them through. They didn't deserve to find me in a drunken stupor, usually lying down on some curb around the area where I had asked them to pick me up. They didn't deserve to go to the hospital after another car accident, wondering if I was still alive or not. They didn't deserve to see their son choose alcohol over a "normal life."

I vividly recall my mom crying uncontrollably and telling me that I was going to lose everything—my wife, my kids, and my job if I kept up the drinking pace I was at. I literally laughed in her face. I remember T. C. telling me at least a hundred times that I needed to slow down or stop completely. She even offered to stop drinking herself to support me. Again, I thought that was funny and laughed it off. The thing I most remember is my daughter Sarah begging me not to go out one night because she knew that I was going to drink. I promised her that I was not going to drink. Of course, I came home at 5 a.m.—hammered. Sad.

Sobriety puts a lot of shit in perspective. I am truly sorry to my parents, my sister, my ex-wife, and, most importantly, my kids for choosing drinking over them for so many years. None of them deserved that. I can't take back those years. I wish I had made better decisions earlier in my life. But while you are going through the drinking years, it is so difficult to think differently. The alcohol consumes you so much that it seems there really is no other choice. Clearly, there are tons of choices you can make in your life, but once that alcohol has you in its clutches, it does not want to let you go.

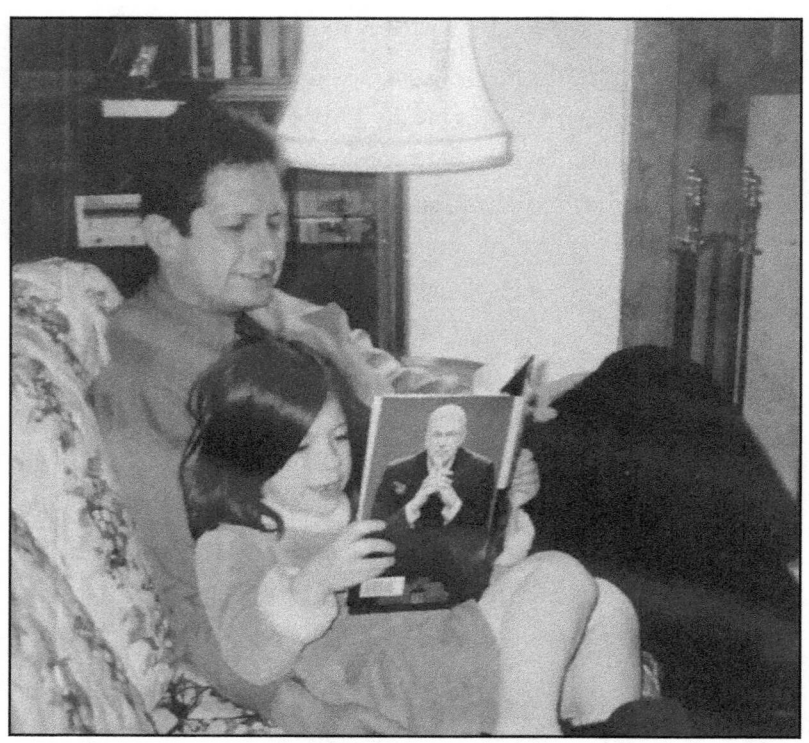

I regret not having more moments like this—reading a book with Isabelle.

I KNOW WHAT IT FEELS LIKE

I KNOW what it feels like . . .

I KNOW what it feels like to be terrified that I will not be able to drink again.

I KNOW what it feels like to be arrested as a direct result of my drinking.

I KNOW what it feels like to be in jail as a direct result of my drinking.

I KNOW what it feels like to see the look of worry in my parent's eyes when they wonder whether I am alive or not because of my drinking.

I KNOW what it feels like to think that there is no way I can stop drinking because it is my personality and I will never be able to have fun again.

I KNOW what it feels like to think: I am not *that* bad.

I KNOW what it feels like to be truly disgusted with myself that I cannot stop drinking.

I KNOW what it feels like to avoid people who think that I have a drinking problem because I know the truth and I am not ready to deal with it.

I KNOW what it feels like to watch my kids beg me to stay home and play with them instead of going out drinking.

I KNOW what it feels like to work extra hard in the entire morning and do chores around the house just so I could have a free afternoon (and night) of drinking.

I KNOW what it feels like to embarrass my children because I was drunk at a kid's event.

I KNOW what it feels like to have a wife have enough of my drinking and want a divorce.

I KNOW what it feels like to only be able see your kids once a week and every other weekend because of my drinking.

I KNOW what it feels like to be escorted out of a job that I loved when I was drunk.

I KNOW what it feels like to be in many car accidents when I was drunk.

I KNOW what it feels like to despise watching my parents drink and watch how they changed personalities under the influence.

I KNOW what it feels like to lay awake in the morning trying to piece together the night before and pray that I didn't say or do anything so stupid that I would get in major trouble.

I KNOW what it feels like to talk shit about other people with drinking problems in order to protect myself and deflect.

I KNOW what it feels like to have this indescribable feeling of despair that came over me when I realized I was an alcoholic—and that every time I tried to do something about it, I failed.

I KNOW what it feels like . . .

But there is hope.

I ALSO KNOW WHAT IT FEELS LIKE TO BE SOBER.

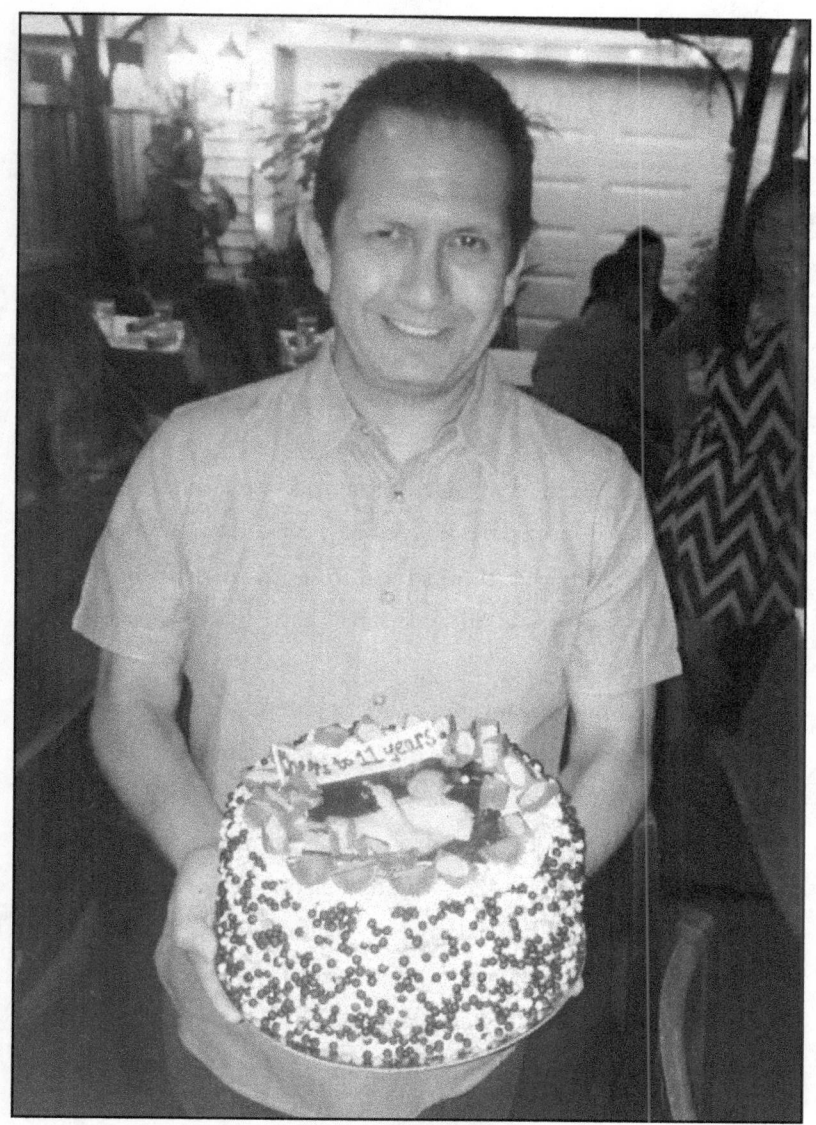

Happy Sobriety to me!

FINAL THOUGHTS

AS I AM writing this, I have been sober for sixteen years. Drinking crosses my mind on a daily basis. I feel like I will never be able to escape it. I wear my sobriety like a badge of honor. I know how difficult it is to get and, more importantly, stay sober. I have dreams (nightmares, really) about drinking that seem so real to me at times. When I wake up and discover that it was just a dream, I have an unbelievable sense of relief.

I am terrified of breaking my sobriety streak. I am very scared to hurt my family and friends. I have talked about sobriety and alcoholism for so long, and now I have written a book about it. As I have stated before, getting sober is such a mental mind fuck. I have to constantly train my mind into believing that alcohol will hurt me in such a way that it will most likely kill me. I know full well what I am capable of. Those stories you just read were not conjured out of thin air. As much as I glorified drinking and laughed out loud at the crazy situations drinking put me in, deep down inside, I know that it was bad for me and I know how serious the consequences were for me.

I have spent the last sixteen years of my life trying to make amends to those whom I hurt while I was drinking. My parents, my children, and my ex-wife are right on top of that list. The longer that I remain sober, the stronger my convictions are to make things right with those I hurt. It is like a vicious circle—but in a good way.

Sobriety has no time limit. It is never too early or too late in your life to start. My recovery started when I was forty-one years old. My daughter Isabelle started her recovery at nineteen years old. There is no right or wrong time. Some people never figure it out. Life is so wonderful without drinking for me—and I can only speak for myself. I cannot get inside anyone else's mind or body. Alcoholism is such a personal thing. I can only share my experiences and hope that at least one person can learn from me.

Today, I do not have to check my phone to see who I called or texted in a drunken state. I am not terrified of walking into work and wondering if anyone can smell my breath. I don't have to use double doses of mouthwash after I brush my teeth. I can call up my kids and ask them if they want to go to lunch or dinner and know I can drive them there and back home. I can stand up in front of a group of people and confidently tell a story without needing alcohol. I can still engage with my friends without the need to drink. I can enjoy any type of event without drinking. I never would have thought any of those things were possible.

I wish I could tell you that sobriety has led the way for me to be the financial success that I have always wanted to be—and that I have several houses and that I go on multiple vacations a year and that I have met the love of my life and that I will live happily ever after. That is simply not true. I do not have money. I can barely pay my mortgage on my condo. I go on zero vacations a year. I am single and sometimes very lonely.

But I do have the one thing that nobody can ever take away from me. I have my sobriety, and I have the ability to talk to people about helping them with their problem with drinking. I know exactly where they have been, and I know exactly where they are going. Hopefully, I can add just a little bit of knowledge and experience to help them stop if they want to.

Every time I look in the mirror these days, it is to see if my hair is properly combed; it is not to question what I am doing with my life. That feels pretty damn good.

My kids are probably so tired of hearing this saying from me, but it is so true and it will never get old in my eyes:

"Wealth in this world is not based on how much you have but rather on how much you give."

I am extremely proud of my sobriety, and I am extremely scared of my sobriety. It is nothing that I will ever take for granted. My sobriety is everything to me, and I understand the value of it.

I hope I helped you.

IN MEMORY OF MY PARENTS

Both of my parents passed away during the writing of this book. Those events truly broke my heart. I have dedicated this book to my parents. I have attached two eulogies that were read by two friends of mine at each service (I apologize in advance for any stories that have already been covered in the book):

MOM:

Hello everybody, my name is Erica Tan. I am a good friend of Eddie Arana, who is the son of Aida. He wrote this knowing that he would not be able to get through this without breaking down, so he asked me to read this. There are going to be some funny moments in this speech, and he didn't want them ruined by constant and unnecessary weeping. So, from now on, I will act and talk as if I am Eddie.

I met my mom in 1963 in San Francisco, California, when she gave birth to me. We lasted in San Francisco for all of about six months before we moved to Chicago. Thank you very much, Mom, for this move to Chicago. I cannot stand heat, humidity, and water, so I am sure I would have been miserable in California.

My first real memory of my mom's kindness was in the seventies when we lived at 7227 North Damen in Chicago's North Side. I had friends who played baseball at Potawatomi Park. I was not very good, and I had told my mom that I wished I were good at baseball. Since my dad had to work six days a week, my mom played catch with me in front of our house for hours on end. She actually had a great arm. I remember that when other kids would walk by, I would try to hide my glove and would tell my om to quit throwing the ball to me. I guess I was ashamed.

When my dad came home from work at Binks Manufacturing Co. in Franklin Park, he would always have a fantastic home-cooked meal waiting for him. Typically, it was a steak and rice and a salad. He liked his steak rare. My mom's rice was always great with the perfect amount of oil and garlic and not too clumpy or too wet. I am still searching for somebody who can cook rice like that. My ex-wife, T. C., got the recipe from my mom and had tried on many occasions, but she just couldn't get it quite right. My mom once told me that she purposely left out one of the ingredients so it would not be perfect. I'm just kidding about that. My mom would never do a bad thing to anybody. She was a living saint.

After high school, a lot of my friends were very anxious to go away and have that "college experience" away from home. That thought never even crossed my mind. I went to DePaul University and lived at home. I loved it. I had the best food in the world cooked for me every night, and I had a great family life. I never really realized how important that truly was to me until recently—and my mom and dad were the reasons for it. My mom instilled in me a desire to do the right thing at all times. I disappointed my mom on so many occasions in my life. I am truly sorry, Mom. But you were the best possible role model growing up, and I hope to pass that on to my children, and I hope they pass it on to their children.

Sometimes, I used to go out and maybe have one or two drinks. I would often call my parents to have them pick me up from whatever corner I happened to be stranded on. My dad would pull up in his green Toronado. My mom would be in the back seat and would let me have the front seat. She would always have a full meal waiting for me IN THE CAR. I mean a rare T-bone steak with a side of rice with corn in it, a salad with Italian dressing, and either a Mott's apple juice or a Welch's grape juice, as well as a Curious George stuffed animal. Do you realize how hard it is to eat a steak dinner in a moving car? That is the type of person she was. She would do anything for her children. I know a lot of people say they would do anything for their children, but my mom and dad really lived that way.

When I was married, we were putting an addition on to our house in Park Ridge. We needed a place to stay for six months. So, me, my T. C., and our kids Sarah, little Eddie, and Isabelle went to live with my parents at 5251 West Argyle. What a glorious time that was for everybody. Home-cooked meals every night. Free babysitting. Free rent. We couldn't have asked for more. Looking back on those days, the real value of that time was that my kids got to spend time with their grandmother, whom they affectionately refer to as Lita, which is short for abuelita in Spanish. They still talk about how they loved staying there and going to the park and going on walks and just spending good-quality family time together.

My parents would do their banking at Chase Bank in Park Ridge. My dad would deposit his check there on a weekly basis. He doesn't believe in direct deposit. Of course, my mom would always be by his side. One of the female bank officers there recently asked me how my mom and dad were doing. She said the people at the bank would refer to my parents as Romeo and Juliet. I think that was a perfect description for them. They were always together, and they would always be holding hands. Relationships like that just do not exist anymore. I know my dad is going to miss her more than anybody can imagine. That was his girl, and he never let her go, and he will love her forever.

Goodbye, Mom. I am not ashamed anymore, and I love you from the bottom of my heart.

DAD:

Good evening. My name is John Moran. I am a fringe friend of Eddie Arana. I apologize that I am a slightly less handsome and taller version of Eddie. He asked me to read this speech to you because he was afraid that he would not be able to get through it without breaking down. So, from now on, I will just read this as if I am Eddie.

My sister, Virginia, and I were in charge of cleaning out my parent's house at 5251 West Argyle in Jefferson Park. This was about eight months ago when they were transitioning to their move to the Norwood Crossing nursing home in Norwood Park. I would go to Argyle every day for a couple of months and sift through their personal belongings to either save them for storage or throw them out or donate them to Goodwill. I was scared to find anything embarrassing that would have painted my dad or my mom in a different light than what I had known them by. I am glad to report that except for a couple of digital scales used to weigh cocaine and marijuana, I found nothing incriminating. I found so many letters and cards that my dad had written my mom throughout the years. There were cards and letters for every holiday imaginable, and some were written for no reason at all. My mom had kept every one of those. I had to rent a separate storage locker just for those letters. Hopefully, they can be sold on Ebay for a nice profit someday.

It is no secret that my dad loved my mom more than anything else in this world. It truly was a love story for the ages. They were married for almost sixty years. Whenever they were together in public, my dad would always make sure he was holding her hand. He wanted the whole world to know that this was his girl. He would always walk on the traffic side of the sidewalk when they were walking together. He would open the car door for her. He would open every door for her. He didn't start eating until my mom had sat down and started eating first. He would introduce her to everybody before he introduced himself to a group. He would always make sure she was safe from harm's way. He was so respectful and kind to my mom, even up to her last day on earth. They don't make gentlemen like that anymore. God really out-did himself with my dad.

My dad did not believe in direct deposit. He was old school like that. He liked to go to the bank and deposit his paycheck himself. He would always take my mom with him on his weekly trips to the Chase Bank in Park Ridge, which happened to be the same bank that I used. The bank employees had nicknamed my parents "Romeo and Juliet." They loved to see the sweet couple who would come in always holding hands with big smiles on their faces. Whenever a bank employee found out that they were my parents, they would go on and on about how wonderful they were and what a love story they were witnessing.

My dad had a world-class sense of humor, and everybody who knew him even a little bit was aware of that. One of my dad's favorite dishes was steak and rice. My mom made the best rice and cooked a great steak. He liked his meat rare. He always told me to "error rare," which meant that once a piece of meat has been overcooked, there is nothing you can do to save it. However, if a piece of meat has been under-cooked, you can always put it back and save the steak. Therefore, if you are going to make an error, make sure that it is on the rare side.

One evening, my mom was preparing my dad a typical steak and rice meal with a bowl of soup. Before she took the soup out to the dining room, I thought it would be funny to empty a bottle of Tabasco into my Dad's soup so I could see his reaction. My mom begged me not to do it, but I convinced her that it would be hilarious and that he would be fine. That bowl had to have been half soup and half hot sauce. I have no idea how anybody could have survived eating it. My mom served him the soup, and I made sure I sat down next to him so I could have the best view of him writhing in pain and get a good laugh out of it. He proceeded to take four or five spoonsful of the soup. He had no reaction. I was floored. How was this even possible? I saw him finish the entire bowl of soup with zero reaction. I was so disappointed. My prank had failed. As I was walking away in disappointment, my dad called me back with a big smile on his face and said, "Hey Eddie, I noticed that soup had a little bite to it, didn't it?" He knew what I had done. He just didn't want me to have the satisfaction of seeing his anguish. That was the kind of relationship that we had. He was the wizard. I could never outdo him.

My dad worked for Sante Fe Railroad in San Francisco around 1960. My mom also worked there as a secretary. My dad was always infatuated with her and tried everything he could in order to date her. On one particular morning, my mom's boss had asked her to take dictation for a speech that he had to make later that evening. My mom confided in my dad that she was very nervous about the dictation because she didn't know English very well, and she felt that he spoke very fast and she would not be able to transcribe his words in a timely and cohesive manner. My dad assured her that everything would be okay.

My mom's boss called her into his office and began to read his speech to her for her to transcribe. He spoke for about fifteen minutes, and then she left his office and sat back down at her desk. My dad approached my mom about ten minutes later and noticed she was struggling with the speech and was visibly upset. He threw a manila envelope on her desk. She opened up the envelope, and it was the speech that she was supposed to transcribe. It was a six-page document in perfect English—probably better than what her boss had actually said. The door was slightly open when her boss was making his speech, and my dad had overheard it and taken the dictation himself at his desk and written and prepared the speech in less than ten minutes. It was grammatically perfect, and every word was spelled correctly. This was way before spell-check even existed. He never asked for a thank you. That was the kind of person he was.

My dad used to take me to many Cubs games at Wrigley Field. We would take the train and get off at Addison and make our way to the ticket window. My dad would ask the ticket attendant what he had available for today's game. Then he would strategically show a little extra money than what the tickets cost—and he would have the tickets in his hand. I would always ask where the seats were located and my dad would never tell me. We would get into the ballpark, and the usher would take our tickets and walk us to our seats. We would always start rather high up in the stadium and continue to go lower and lower and lower, and we always ended up within the first five rows near home plate—the best seats in the house. I always asked him, "How did you do that?" He would just smile and asked me if I wanted a hot dog. Being at a Cubs game with my dad was the best feeling imaginable to me. I thought I was the luckiest kid in the world. I didn't think life could get any better than that.

My dad and I thoroughly enjoyed the Chicago Bulls championship during the Michael Jordan years. I had season tickets and would always take my dad to all of the playoff games. We missed a few Christmas and Easter dinners because we had to go the United Center to watch the Bulls play.

We were at one Bulls NBA Finals game in the nineties, and my Dad had noticed that I hadn't been myself the entire day. During the game, he asked me what the problem was. I told him that I had gotten into a disagreement with this girl whom I really liked at work, and I felt horrible about it. She was going out of town that day for a vacation with her girlfriends in the Bahamas, and her flight was in a few hours. Once the game was over, we got into my dad's car, and he made a stop at Nordstrom's. He told me to wait in the car. He came back with a package that I thought was a present for my mom. Then he asked me what airline she was flying to the Bahamas. We drove to the airport, and my dad gave me the package, which contained a monkey stuffed animal, and he told me to give it to the girl and make sure everything was okay before she got on her flight. He knew exactly what I needed to do to make things right. I ended up marrying the girl whom I gave that monkey to. My dad knew how to treat and respect women more than any man I have ever met in my life.

Later on in his life, my dad was an interpreter for the State of Illinois Circuit Court of Cook County. He made many friends at that job. The majority of comments from his coworkers since my dad's passing have been related to his being a complete gentleman, his love for my mom, his being a genius, his amazing tie collection, and the shininess of his shoes. Nobody had a bad word to say about my dad. He could also do a *New York Times* crossword puzzle in about four minutes. Does anybody know how hard a *New York Times* crossword puzzle is? And also, are you aware that the puzzles get harder and harder as the week goes by—Monday being the easiest up until Friday, which is the hardest? The Sunday *New York Times* crossword is the big daddy of all the crossword puzzles. My dad needed at least fifteen minutes to complete that one. Oh, and he never used a pencil. He would always use a pen, and he never needed Wite-Out because he never made a mistake. If you did use a pencil with an eraser on it, he would consider that cheating.

I cannot imagine a better role model to have growing up than my dad. He set me an impossible bar to measure up to. He was small in stature, but he was a giant to me. I love you, Dad, from the bottom of my heart, and I miss you so much already.

Goodbye, Romeo. Go be with Juliet. She has been waiting for you. I have everything under control here. You don't need to worry anymore. Rest in peace.

UPDATE

July 15, 2020

HERE IS MY post on Facebook that day:

I am 16 years sober today. Yes, it is a big deal. I am very proud of myself. I want the entire world to know about it. Yes, I am extremely proud to call myself an alcoholic. I am not ashamed or afraid or embarrassed to use that term—being an alcoholic was the worst thing that ever happened to me, and it turned out to be the best thing that ever happened to me.

Waking up today to the text pictured below from my daughter, Isabelle Arana, who is 18 months sober, makes everything that I do and talk about and write about worth it for me. She is 20 years old and is on the same journey as I am. She is very proud also.

This has not been the easiest year for me or my family, but I held on to the most important thing in my life—my sobriety. Without my sobriety, I have nothing. Thank you everybody for helping to keep me sober. I can mark another red X on my calendar today.

If you are struggling with drinking or drugging, I feel your pain. I am not you, but I know you. I cannot feel what you are feeling, but I have felt those exact same feelings of fear and desperation and helplessness. It is possible to stop, and it doesn't matter how old you are or how bad you are. I want to help one person. Is it you? #IceWaterPlease

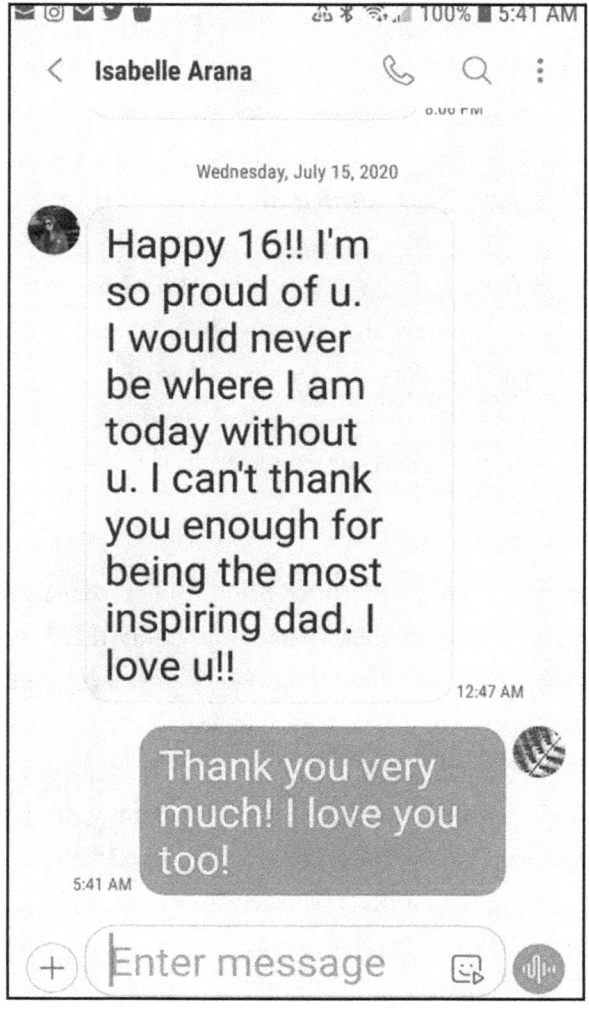